THE NATURE OF
BREATHING

Dedicated to my daughter Beth, who
is my best and most challenging teacher

THE NATURE OF
BREATHING

Jenny Beeken

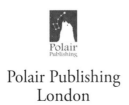

Polair Publishing
London

First published October 2021

British Library Cataloguing-in-Publication Data
A catalogue reference for this book is
obtainable from the British Library

ISBN 978-1-905398-55-3

Printed in the Czech Republic
with the assistance of Akcent Media

CONTENTS

ACKNOWLEDGMENTS

MY FIRST idea for a book on breathing came from a walk with Rose Thorn, where she told me about James Nestor's book BREATH. We had quite a discussion. So I read the book with much interest and focus, especially on where he investigates yoga practices, realizing that I could go on from the yoga that he references in it to expand into specific practices that will support and transform how we breathe. So thank you very much to James for the ways in which he has opened up my mind. And thank you Rose for the recommendation.

I thank my editor and publisher, Colum Hayward, for his faith in the book and his support in the ideas and the writing of it and everything especially the enormous time commitment.

Great thanks to Murray Nettle for her delightful, instructive drawings – anatomical and postural – for her diligence in getting them just right, and also for her photos.

Cryn Horn's section on *yoga nidra* is a great addition. So thank you, Cryn. And thank you to my students for their contributions. Bridget Whitehead has written on peripheral vision and given much help in discussions and research. Thank you, Bridget.

Tina Moxon, Lisa Christensen, Bridget Whitehead and Jared Bell were enthusiastic subjects for photos and photographers too. Thank you all. And thank you Sarah Robinson and Ken Bell, my diligent proofreaders.

A thank you to Jeremy Hayward for photographing the monks, to Bruce Clarke for his wonderful shot of interlocking trees, and the many other photographers not individually mentioned here.

Thank you to the Cittaviveka Community, Ajahn Ahimsako and Ajahn Gavesako for their support in checking the Buddha's teachings that are included. Also thanks to Sihanado Bhikkhu and Cagadhammo Bhikkhu for their walking meditations.

'Breathing is the essence of yoga.
Breathe naturally without forcing.
No pressure, no disturbance, nothing should interfere with the simple, tide-like movement of our lungs as we breathe in and out.
After a while, if we are paying attention, we will find that the last
three vertebrae closest to the ground begin to receive life. The energy
running along the back of the spine from its base to the top of the
head increases in power, making the spine alive and strong.
What is important is the regularity of the breath. Do not try to take
long breaths, their length will slowly increase. It is only a question
of time.'
Vanda Scaravelli, AWAKENING THE SPINE

'I vividly remember my first day of monk school…. I noticed a
child monk – he can't have been more than ten years old – teaching
a group of five-year-olds. He had a great aura about him, the poise
and confidence of an adult.
"'What are you doing?" I asked.
"'We just taught their first class ever", he said, then asked me,
"'What did you learn in your first day of school?"
"'I started to learn the alphabet and numbers. What did they
learn?"
"'The first thing we teach them is how to breathe."
"'Why?" I asked.
"'Because the only thing that stays with you from the moment you're
born until the moment you die is your breath. All your friends,
your family, the country you live in, all of that can change. The one
thing that stays with you is your breath.'"
Jay Shetty, THINK LIKE A MONK

Introduction

*'On rising, face the Sun, if possible before an open window
(which should have been open all night). Stand erect so that you
are correctly polarised, with the spine straight.
'As you inhale, centre your whole concentration on the Sun; as
you breathe, realize that you are breathing not only air but very
life-atoms (prana in Sanskrit) into your being. Raise your arms
(to the side) as you breathe in, and then as you breathe out let
your arms fall slowly.'*

White Eagle

ARE YOU aware of how you breathe? Are you aware of any
changes in your breathing as you go about your day? Are you
aware of connecting with the world around you?

There has been much said about the changes that have
been brought about by the lockdowns set up to contain the
pandemic of Covid-19 in 2020/21. One of the main effects
seems to me to have been to encourage people to go outside
into nature – whether walking, gardening, or simply appreci-
ating nature. All these activities have been taken up far more.
For myself, I go outside every morning to do as the teacher
White Eagle advises in the paragraph above.

So are we now leading a more natural life and is that helping
us to breathe more naturally and vice versa? Has the pandemic
changed the world? I thought it would at the beginning, that
we would care more for each other and take care of ourselves
more – caring in the process for the animal kingdom, nature,
and the world that we inhabit immediately around us, as well

as the whole planet. Now, as I write, we are making the very decisions that will shape life to come. To breathe with more awareness of how our breath moves through our body may be the best resolution we can make.

Why Breathing?

Modern life gives us lots of reminders that we tend to ignore. When my daughter was living in Australia a few years back, I visited Uluru, which is the correct aboriginal name for Ayers Rock, and the name that's now used in Australia. We had an aboriginal guide taking us around, explaining the sacredness of Uluru to his people. He challenged all those on the tour by what he reminded us of – with the charge that we fly around the world, visiting places of interest that we think should be visited – and then fly on somewhere else to take yet more photos! And then we rush on yet again.

We learnt that Australian aboriginal people consider that they are born to a certain place in order to take care of the land there – and that is simply what they do (unless their land is interfered with by invaders). Maybe we could take some wisdom from them and stop rushing around, and be with where we are now? Awareness of how we breathe would certainly enable us to do that more.

More recently I heard a discussion on BBC Radio 4 designed to give the message that unless we address climate change, animal welfare, the destruction of nature (in particular its rain forests and other natural habitats) and with it the stress we put ourselves under in order to have a good life, we will go on getting pandemics and they will change everything for us!

It's an alarming thought.

And I expect that like me you've watched Greta Thunberg – maybe on the BBC series, 'A year to change the world'. The programme is about her at the age of sixteen, travelling around Canada and on down the American West Coast. Her very youth symbolizes our greatest hope that we may be able to stop the destruction of the planet, by changing direction. On the West Coast, she found alarming evidence of drastic events that indicate what may become of those who are in the poorer and most affected parts of the world, while others go on destroying the planet: felling trees, using fossil fuel and living as though we are not in a crisis. The programme at the very least made me feel that I would not easily get on a plane again.

Another thing we have come to recognize is that air quality has an absolutely radical effect on our health. London, for instance, has had to introduce an 'ultra-low emission zone' just to make sure that large numbers of its citizens do not die of exhaust fumes. There has recently been a well-publicized case:

> 'A coroner has called for a change in the law after air pollution led to the death of a nine-year-old girl. Ella-Adoo-Kissi-Debrah, who lived near the South Circular in Lewisham, southeast London, died in 2013. An inquest found that air pollution made a 'material contribution' to her death.
>
> *https://www.bbc.co.uk/uk-London-England-56801794*
> *(April 2021)*

I was brought up in Lewisham, south London. Sixty or seventy years ago it was like a country village, with a great street market where I would do my grandmother's shopping, and an old-fashioned grocer where all the staff knew your name and served you individually. They knew exactly what my mother and grandmother liked and wrapped it all in brown paper. The air was very clear there then!

Cities all around the world are having to do the same sort of things as London with its 'ULEZ' (Ultra-low emission zone). There may well be a connection between air pollution and the severity of Covid-19.

It all adds up to one thing: we have to change.

Making Changes

Breathing is a very good place to begin that change, as it is so fundamental to us and is very linked to the mind. Habitual ways of breathing link to habitual ways of thinking. Moreover, the majority of us have an unnatural breathing pattern. To quote the author of a recent book on breathing, we are 'the worst breathers in the animal kingdom.'*

Any long-term change in how well we breathe will have an effect on our posture, the health of our body and mind, and on our mind-patterns – and vice versa. It will go on to affect our desires and our fears – which in turn are at the root of our over-consumption. Because of the consciousness that goes with it, it will even bring better balance to the carbon dioxide emissions problem – or at the very least it could develop in us the awareness and sensitivity to play our part in controlling climate change. I will return to this at the end of the book.

I have noticed that when my mind is very busy, my breathing is extremely shallow. I feel as though I am hardly breathing at all. If this busy attitude changes, our posture changes, and as

*See James Nestor, BREATH (Penguin Life, 2020). I shall draw on the information in this groundbreaking book quite frequently, going on from it to give more information and practices that address how we breathe and how it is linked to how we live.

our breathing changes, our mind changes.

In order to make any difference to the patterns we've built up, we need at first to become aware of our breath as it comes in and goes out, and particularly to notice whether we are breathing through our nose – which is the organ designed for the breath – or through our mouths. Really, this is as easy as it sounds but it can be enormously challenging for us, as it touches deeply-held habits, possibly the habits of several generations.

Just as we copy our parents and those who care for us – their posture, ways of moving, speaking, lifestyle, careers, opinions – or rebel against them, of course, which can be on a very subtle level – we also copy breathing patterns. A number of people I have spoken to can remember noticing how their parents breathed. It is natural to copy what you remember.

In many years of yoga teaching, I have been very aware of those with high blood pressure breathing predominantly through the mouth, with the head tilted up slightly to relieve the pressure on the carotid artery in the neck. My mother was one who breathed a great deal through her mouth, and had extremely high blood pressure. Her doctors could not believe that she did not feel very ill with it. I think she got used to it over a long time, probably at least since her teenage years, when she felt deeply anxious, spending days and nights in air-raid shelters in London during the second world war. She also suffered severe depression and anxiety over many years.

Is there a link between her high blood pressure, her depression and her breathing? Current research would suggest that there most definitely is. This book will show that there is a way forward, and that it is not a hard one. The best way of breathing comes completely naturally to us. You don't have to be a yoga student to get help from this book, but at the heart of it is the absolutely natural pursuit of *pranayama*, or breath awareness. Sometimes *pranayama* is translated as 'control of the breath' – but control implies a kind of violence, and that's the opposite of what this book proposes. At the beginning of chapter 4, a quotation from a modern introduction to the ancient yoga text, Patanjali's Sutras on Yoga makes it clear that 'awareness' is the right word rather than 'control'. There are what seem like weird and wonderful ways of breathing encouraged in yoga practice, and many of them, too. However, what appears weird in our breathing does occur naturally in different circumstances of our daily life, and therefore the so called 'techniques' are actually adaptations to those circumstances. With that awareness *pranayama* can be practised more naturally and therefore more easily. It is this absolutely natural approach I hope you will find helpful in these pages.

Hopefully you will find here the most appropriate practice for you – one which progressively brings you health, vitality and balance within the natural world.

Chapter 1 : Breathing Naturally

Mouth and Nose Breathing

THERE IS evidence from ancient skulls that our ancestors, the early members of the species *homo sapiens,* would have breathed through their nostrils. Perhaps you can see in the photo – which is a reconstruction from archaeological finds* – that the nostrils are very wide, as is the whole skull, and the mouth is closed. By contrast I have noticed in a great many photos of people today, in advertizing and in the media, that they have their mouths open. This means that they would inevitably be

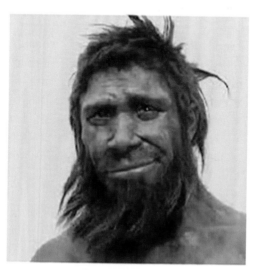

Reconstruction from an ancient skull showing the wide nostrils and jaw and a broad closed mouth

breathing through the mouth, at least partially, whereas you will notice that in the picture of the Native American mother and child on p. 21, they have their mouths firmly closed.

When considering how we might breathe more easily, naturally, deeply, we need to begin by taking a look at what opening we breathe through. It soon becomes clear how much we actually breathe through our mouths as a societal norm. Since the industrial revolution and the pollution it has brought with it, mouth breathing has hugely increased among humans. But breathing through the mouth is largely unknown in other mammals except in special circumstances. A dog will pant, but more to cool itself than to get more air. It has become progressively more of a challenge to breathe through our noses, especially since we live life in a perpetual rush.

There is a theory that mouth breathing actually started many thousands of years ago on the plains of Africa. First *homo sapiens* developed the opposable thumb, from the rotation of the forearm bones (the radius and ulna) so that he could make and use weapons such as bows and arrows or spears. Then language developed, and the brain started getting bigger. Humans were then able to start thinking about taking over the world and have progressively concluded that they had 'dominion over nature' – even to the extent of claiming they were told they were its masters by God! Maybe that arrogance in itself made our brains that much bigger. Anyway, we then started cooking meat and mashing food to make it softer and easier and more palatable to eat. And in return we have dental problems and nasal obstructions.

All three of the developments mentioned (the enlarged brain, nasal breathing and chewing less) caused the face to narrow, the mouth to get smaller and the nose to protrude. This has not happened to any other mammal. Other mammals' nasal passages are much broader and their mouths much bigger; and they have to tear and chew their food, whether it is meat, grass or trees.

That's how they are in nature, anyway. What happens when mammals such as dogs are interfered with by selective breathing is very different: inbred dogs such as pugs and French bulldogs have nasal obstructions that gives them a lot of problems.

Indigenous Africans, Native Americans and the people of many such cultures do have wider faces and more open nostrils and do not have the dental problems or nasal obstruction that the western 'civilization' has developed.

To see research on this you can study online the Morton collection of skulls at the University of Pennsylvania Museum of Archeology and Anthropology – and the work that Dr Marianna Evans, an orthodontist and dental researcher, has conducted on these hundreds of skulls quite recently. You may be alarmed to discover that Samual Morton first collected these skulls in the early nineteenth century in order to show that the skulls of the African and indigenous cultures showed an inferiority in brain development as a justification for slavery. He of course failed, and subsequently the work of Evans and others has shown that the subjects in the collection were much healthier then, with the wider face and more open nostrils, and that thus they did not need to breathe through their mouths.

Mouth breathing is not natural, but it is very common in Western civilization for many reasons. Increasing levels of pollution cause constriction in the sinuses, nose, trachea and lungs, and as a result it becomes much easier – even necessary from time to time – to breathe through the mouth. This then increases the restrictions in the nasal passages further, until eventually it becomes habitual. This can be from infancy if a baby sleeps in a stuffy room with no ventilation.

From then on, entire lack of awareness of one's breath takes over, which makes it feel natural and easy to continue breathing through the mouth, so that many people do not realize that that is what they are doing. Later, diseases and infections of the lungs and the whole respiratory system may occur, causing constriction in the throat, nostrils, and the windpipe (trachea). These in turn make it feel imperative to breathe through the mouth.

The problem is then that the infection increases, because there is no cleansing of the air, which is the job of the nose. The nose has tiny hairs called *cilia* that cleanse, warm, purify and pressurize the air ready for the lungs. This is important for the capacity of the lungs and for the diffusion of oxygen and carbon dioxide.

Breathing, unlike most other functions of the body, can be automatic and unconscious, or it can be conscious. We can be so preoccupied with getting on with our day that we simply forget that we are breathing at all. Automatically we take the easy option – and take short breaths through the mouth. This means we breathe much faster and tend to use the top part of the lungs more. Doing this is detrimental to the function of the lungs and heart and circulatory system, for it increases the heart rate, reduces the amount of oxygen transported into the blood and all around the body, and affects the sympathetic nervous system, increasing stress and anxiety and promoting depression.

The Influence of Posture

Another very crucial element in breathing is our posture, especially when we are sitting. If the spine is collapsed down and back into a chair – or, even more, into a sofa or armchair – the diaphragm cannot move to take the breath in fully to the bottom of the lungs (see chapter 2, which is about our anatomy). So very short, superficial breaths tend to be taken through the mouth and into the very top of the chest only. I'll return to this later.

It isn't just when we believe we are relaxing that this happens. If the lumbar spine is collapsed back then the neck vertebrae (cervical spine) also collapse back, and so the head drops forward, feeling too heavy for the neck. This is typical 'computer posture'.

The chin then tucks into the chest and the throat closes up (don't worry: chapter 3 offers yoga postures to remedy this!). The closed throat severely restricts the passage of air into the lungs and again we feel the unconscious need to take short sharp breaths through the mouth, much too fast for the natural breathing rate, and only then take the breath into the top part of the lungs.

If the lumbar area (the small of the back) has become weak and collapsed on the pelvis from sitting as described for long periods of time, then when we stand or try to sit straight the lumbar area pushes forward and collapses down on the pelvis. This in turn makes the neck vertebrae collapse – that is, curve forward – so that the head and chin go up and back. Then the mouth opens and so mouth breathing is much more likely. (Again, go to chapter 3 for postures to change your day-to-day posture.)

Understanding this, it is amazing that we are alive, isn't it? – but at times we can feel only half alive. Is the way we breathe the reason? How many of us do feel tired, overdone, stressed, half alive? What would happen if we were to address how we are breathing? And understand how we could breathe more naturally? These are the big questions that I would like to address in this little book.

More on Mouth Breathing

There are other problems with mouth breathing. It encourages air down into the digestive system, creating difficulties in digesting food, and so increases flatulence and constipation. Also, the nervous system is agitated in mouth breathing, which increases anxiety and stress and those in turn increase the tendency to breathe through the mouth.

The problems are often very evident after running or strong physical exertions – the puffing and panting we tend to go through are largely unnecessary. There is a Jamaican-American

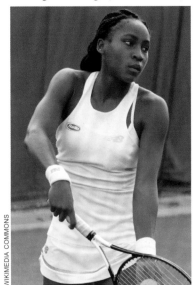

WIKIMEDIA COMMONS

sprinter named Sanya Richards-Ross who trained herself to breathe only through the nose while she ran. She won the 400m Gold in the 2012 Olympics and finished smiling and very calm – quite unlike her competitors. She now trains other runners in nose breathing.* The picture shows a tennis professional at Wimbledon who resolutely breathes through her nose: Coco Gauff.

Nearly two hundred years ago, in America, a young artist left his 'day job' and travelled among the indigenous peoples. He was called George Catlin (1796-1872). In 1862 he published a study called THE BREATH OF LIFE (it was later republished under the title 'Shut your

*See www.yumpu.com/nose-breathingpaysoff

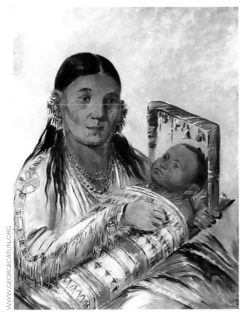

mouth and save your life'). Interestingly, he wrote it after living with American Indian tribes in the 1830s. He describes seeing mothers, after breast feeding was complete, putting their baby down and gently closing his or her lips – and then repeating that if the baby's mouth opened at all while sleeping. In this way they ensured that nose breathing became a natural habit from infancy. Catlin goes on to say:*

'Then when I have seen careful, tender, civilized mothers covering their babies' heads, sleeping in overheated rooms with their little mouths open gasping for breath; and afterwards looked into the multitude and seen the long-lasting results of this incipient stage of education; and have been forcibly struck and shocked by this the results of this habit thus contracted and practised in contravention to natures design.... There is no animal in nature excepting man, who sleeps with the mouth open.

'Too much sleep is said to be destructive to health; but very

*Catlin's whole book is available online: see https://archive.org/details/shutyourmouth.

few persons sleep too much provided they sleep in the right way. Unnatural sleep, which is irritating to the lungs and nervous system, fails to afford that rest which sleep is intended to give, and the longer one lies in it the less will be the enjoyment and length of life. Anyone waking in the morning at their usual hour of arising and finding by the dryness of the mouth, that they have been sleeping with the mouth open, feels fatigued and wishes to go to sleep again; and convinced that their rest has not been good enough,' they are then ready to admit the truth of the statement above.'

It was very much a habit in the Natural American Indian tribes to keep the mouth closed when not eating or talking to stop any germs and infections going into the mouth and then lungs, without the purifying effect of going through the nostrils. It also reduces greatly the strength of the body, deforms the face as the jaw drops and narrows, increasing stress and disease. Native Americans said that 'the air that enters your lungs (through the nostrils) is as different as distilled water is from the water in a frog pond.'

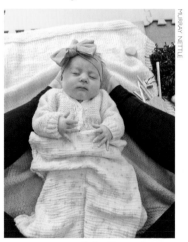

MURRAY NETTLE

Nose Breathing

Having read these strictures, which have made me aware of how much I breathe through my mouth, I have attended mindfully to breathing through my nose, to the ex-

Baby Sienna has her mouth naturally closed

tent of putting a piece of surgical tape over my mouth at night. I have noticed that my head feels clearer: I am more alert. My digestion is much better. I eat more slowly and do not get air into the digestive tract. My nostrils have changed shape: they have opened up and flared out at the sides, so that I can take more air in with each inhalation. Then the air sacs deep in my lungs fill up more efficiently, giving me more energy. This, I understand, is also beneficial for the heart: it is cleansed and so works more efficiently and becomes better regulated.

The exhalation is gentler and fuller. I can walk uphill more easily now, although it was harder at first, when I really had to focus on keeping my mouth shut. I can walk for longer without tiring and stride out more. I wake up more refreshed so do not need so much sleep. I do not wake up with a dry mouth so have probably not been snoring.

I am aware of the cleansing effect of the small hairs mentioned earlier, the cilia in the nostrils that filter out dust, pathogens, allergens and pollen before they reach the throat and lungs. (see chapter 4, on *pranayama* – particularly *kapabalati* (p. 88) to increase the cleansing). Doing this during the Covid-19 respiratory virus has felt very significant. I have wondered if it would even reduce the likelihood of infection.

There are modern researchers who agree wholeheartedly with George Catlin. See, for example, the article 'Mouth breathing and the dentist', by Janice Goodman and Mark Webb on the website, Oral Health. It is especially useful on the importance of nasal breathing – and something which we now discover to be vital is nitric oxide:

'Nasal breathing has been well documented to provide various benefits. The nose is equipped with a complex filtering system which purifies the air we breathe before it enters the lungs. Breathing through the nose during exhalation helps maintain lung volumes and so may indirectly determine arterial oxygenation.

'One of the most important reasons for nasal breathing is … the production of nitric oxide.…

'Although this gas is produced in minute amounts, when it is inhaled through the nose to the lungs, it will follow the airstream to the lower airways and lungs, where it aids in increasing arterial oxygen tension; hence enhancing the lungs' capacity to absorb oxygen.

'Nitric oxide also plays an important role in reducing high blood pressure, maintaining homeostasis, Immune defence and neurotransmission.'

https://www.oralhealthgroup.com/features/
mouth-breathing-physical-mental-emotional-consequences/

Patrick McKeown, in his deep and thorough scientific book THE BREATHING CURE has done a lot of work with children who have developed physical and mental problems, which he connects to mouth breathing. He recommends that they actually put a piece of tape over the mouth for half an hour every day when they are doing something that distracts them, such as watching the television. The effect has been to gradually break the habit of mouth breathing. I felt I needed to do that too!

About twenty years ago, when I first heard of keeping the mouth closed at night with a piece of tape, I thought I could not do that and that I didn't need it. I was not aware of how much I breathed through my mouth. When I tried it, recently, I could not keep the tape there for more than an hour or two. Now I am relatively comfortable with it all night. After about two months of doing it I find it reassuring and helpful. I do not know how long I need to do it for; it is said that it takes as many months to break a habit as the years you have had the habit so that's about five years for me!* It is also making me more aware of how I can sometimes breathe through my mouth in the day – especially when in a hurry, anxious or lacking in awareness.

Being mindful of breathing with the mouth closed, especially when walking, is also very helpful to nose breathing. There is a rhythm to it. Walking in a forest, or as the Japanese describe it, 'Forest Bathing' (one of the reasons for the choice of the cover of this book) you will find that there is an interchange of oxygen and carbon dioxide between you and the trees. This is very cleansing and purifying on the whole respiratory tract, and therefore the circulatory system, so that it revitalizes the mind and body. To be aware of the living, breathing trees and connecting with them really encourages the breath to be natural and easy. Using the imagination helps. The large tall trees in forests in Hampshire, where I used to live, are very uplifting, while the trees in the coastal region of West Wales, where I now am, tend to be much smaller – but then the leaves are much nearer you. In the paradise gardens of Iran, ancient Persia, the trees are put at a lower level than the walkways so that you are at the level of the leaves and flowers as you walk around them enjoying the beautiful aroma and breathing in the fresh air.

Wales also gives me the opportunity for walking by the sea

*An update four months later! I started not using the tape every night in the last month and have felt it more difficult not to breathe through my mouth during the day, especially if walking uphill. So rather than occasionally using it or a few nights a week or for part of the night, I have felt the need to go back to using it every night. As is often stated, old habits are hard to break.

In fact, there is now special tape for the purpose! On YouTube (www. myotape.com) you can see Patrick's daughter, Lauren, modelling it.

with its refreshing layer of ozone, that clears the nostrils and
encourages the lungs to fill.

> 'The forest gives pure air for us to breathe. The forest means
> everything to my tribe, it is our life, our body. We are still the
> same – we still live the same as we have always done – in tune
> with nature – you are welcome to come and visit us to see.
> I am asked why is the climate changing? It's lack of love and
> understanding of each other."
> *Nixiwaka of the Yamanana tribe, Amazon Rain forest, Brazil.*
> *Tedtalks.com*

In your nasal breathing practice, do not give up if there
is congestion in
the nose. This can
be cleared by per-
severance but does
not always feel
easy. A neti pot
can help, where
you pour salted
water through
each nostril (please
see chapter 4, on
yoga practices) as
well as being out-
side a lot. Can
you get into the
habit of going out
first thing in the
morning to greet
the dawn wherever

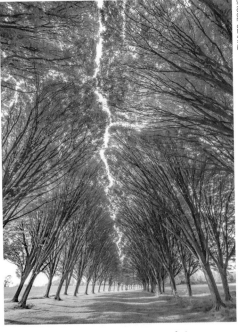
BRUCE CLARKE

These interlocking trees remind me of the arrange-
you are – at least *ment of the alveoli (air sacs) of the lungs (see p. 38)*

for some of the year?

Seeing what I had written, my friend Colum Hayward added:

'Greeting the dawn is more easily done in some seasons and climates than others, but one group that makes a sacred practice of it is the fraternity in Bulgaria founded by the teacher Peter Deunov (1864-1944). His followers stand facing the dawn wherever they can get a clear view of the eastern horizon. They watch as the great red disc comes over that horizon, and raise their right hand in salute as the full disc becomes clear. It is of course dangerous to stare at the sun when it goes over a certain height, but when it is rising the light is so filtered that to gaze at it is regarded as beneficial in itself. The Bulgarian disciple may then say a prayer such as

> *The disciple [of God] has*
> *A heart as pure as a crystal*
> *A mind bright as the sun*
> *A soul vast as the universe*
> *And a spirit as powerful as God*
> *And one with God.*

Peter Deunov is also the creator of the practice known as paneurhythmy, a kind of sacred dance bringing together the influences of the earth and the sky.'

Whatever practice you choose, it is always helpful to find a spot that you can feel comfortable to return to each day. Ideally with bare feet firmly planted on the Earth, honour the sky by lifting the arms and whole upper body. Honour the Earth by taking your hands down on the Earth, and honour yourself, the great Masters and all of humanity, by placing your hands together. This will open out the body and wake up the spine and the diaphragm, which have been rested during sleep.

My daughter lives high up in a London block of flats but she is lucky enough to have a balcony overlooking an amazing and enormous old willow tree in the car park outside. It feels wonderful to greet the tree when I first get up whenever I stay there. It has also woken up her and her flatmate's awareness of nature and how it changes day by day.

So do find your own spot – even if it means a bit of a walk, which is good in itself.

> 'Do not visit your friend's house when you are ill or sick. Do not go to your friend's house when you are unhappy or mad. Stay in the forest, walk among the trees or around the lake and complain to them. Then, when your mind is calm and your heart is free, visit your friends and pay tribute and affection to them.'
>
> *Peter Deunov*

Peter Deunov also made some remarks about our needing to spend some time high up, above the tree line, each year, so that we take in the *prana* that the trees can't reach – a con-

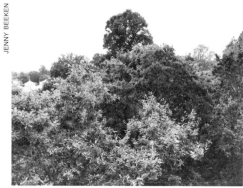

trasting viewpoint to the one where we draw strength from the example of the trees!

The practice of sitting outdoors in the awareness of your breath natu-

From the Kew Gardens Treetop Walkway   rally coming in and going out is not only conducive to nostril breathing but is settling to the mind, feelings and emotions. Again, see chapter 4 for detailed instructions and different breathing for changing states of mind and body.

There may be many ways in which trees will be our salvation, A BBC reporter, Ade Adepitan, recently said in a programme about climate change that planting trees is one of the most effective and cheapest ways of tackling it. The Himalayan nation of Bhutan is actually carbon negative, he pointed out. Seventy per cent of their land is covered in trees; there are very few cars on the road and the number of tourists flying in is very strictly limited. The prime minister is not seeking for economic growth but for the contentment, harmony and health of the people of Bhutan, who follow the teachings of the Lord Buddha.

Balancing the Inhalation and Exhalation

There is much research that shows how common it is for us to breathe quite forcefully in and make some noise doing it, but not to breathe right out. Yet to exhale fully is as important if not more important than a complete inhalation.

In natural breathing, the breath needs to come in silently and go out silently. Then it is not forceful or strained. (Exceptions are two techniques given in the *pranayama* chapter: *kapabalati*, the shining skull breath, and *bastrika*, the bellows breath, also known as fire breath.)

If we concentrate too much on the inbreath, we are tending to over-breathe and to retain too much air and too much oxygen – and then tend to breathe out forcefully but not fully, and through the mouth. Probably the first person to bring this to our attention was a Russian doctor, Konstantin Pavlovich

Buteyko, in the 1950s. His method of extending the exhalation and then holding the breath out was developed specially to help asthma sufferers. His method has helped a great many people, even though it has been criticized by the medical profession as not effective and also for the length of time focused on the exhalation.

As you begin the exhalation practice, it comes more naturally if there is more of a pause at the end of the exhalation rather than a holding (a rather subtle but distinct difference) and a waiting for the breath to find its way in, rather than drawing it in. You do not need to do that; it will happen just by itself. You cannot stop it – the life very much wants to

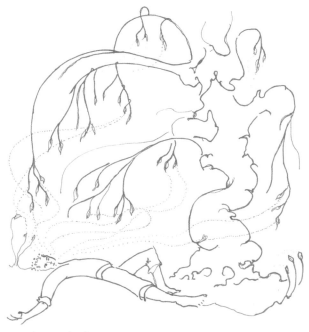

Exchange of gifts: oxygen and carbon dioxide are inhaled and
exhaled in a continuous chain. For our need for carbon dioxide, see pp 43-4

A Practice
of Simply Breathing

This is best practised lying down to start with, but afterwards you can more easily do it standing or sitting. Lie preferably on the floor or outside in nature. If you cannot get on the floor or it's difficult to sit, or you are in a wheelchair, try lifting your legs onto a stool or chair; it will allow the spine to move forward and up more and thus allow the diaphragm to wake up. See the next chapter, on 'How the body works', for the function of the diaphragm.

Bring your eyes to look downwards so that you can focus on your breathing moving in and out. Make sure your mouth is gently and lightly closed.

Do not try to make your breath come in or go out – just notice how you are breathing, for two or three minutes.

Can you feel that your awareness of your breathing pattern will tend to lengthen both the inhalation and the exhalation, without you doing anything?

Go with this movement, focusing for a few breaths on the exhalation – as though you are travelling with it. Does it naturally extend?

Can you pause at the end of the exhalation and wait for the breath to come in of its own accord, so that it is like a wave coming in and then going out?

come in, doesn't it? Then it is more natural and the habit of not breathing right out is gently addressed over time. The length of the exhalation and the pause can be very gradually extended over time too.

An adept in yoga – a true yogi or yogini – when they come to the end of their life and know that they are dying will consciously breathe out and then not breathe in! So you can be aware of how much the life-force wants to come in after a pause and know that there is more for you to experience on this Earth!

What I have noticed about habits is that if you try to break an unwanted habit forcefully and quickly, then it will likely return as soon as you get tired of being forceful. On the other hand, if a habit first comes to your awareness, and then you very gently address and begin to change it and bring that awareness of how you breathe into your daily life and into whatever you are doing, then there is a gradual transformation and more long-lasting change in the unhelpful habit.

I once heard Sri BKS Iyengar describe the breath verbally in this way (the words are from my notes):

> Welcome the inhalation as though it is an old friend, that you have not seen for a long time and are very pleased to see. Then go with the exhalation as though you are going with that friend down the path – a little reluctant to see them go – so that the exhalation is naturally slow and extended.

Feel the effect of doing this. Don't do it for too long, as if you do so there is a tendency to try and make it happen – or to 'go at it'. Rather, it needs regular daily practice until it becomes more of a habit to breathe more easily and naturally.

Chapter 2 : How the Body Works

'There is wisdom to be received from the body, a memory of lightness and simple symmetry from the time when we were forming and moving within a fluid environment. One can regain and recall this sense.

'As we move upward through the spine to discover the rhythm of the lungs, we find more freedom, more connections. We learn to trust the intelligence of the body, particularly those which lead us back to the spine.... The body keeps defining itself; when one part becomes more intelligent other parts change and rearrange themselves.'

Diane Long and Sophy Hoare, NOTES ON YOGA

The Structure of the Respiratory Tract

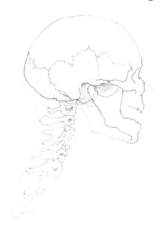

See how the skull is very finely balanced on the vertebrae in the neck

FOUR YEARS ago, I wrote a book called STANDING, SITTING, WALKING, RUNNING in which I wrote at length about the whole posture of the body from the feet upwards, and the action of the diaphragms from that perspective. In fact, I have spent forty-two years seeing the body in that order – and feel that I have really only just come to address the shoulders, neck and head in a way that allows them to move more freely myself. So this time, I am going to start at the top of the body.

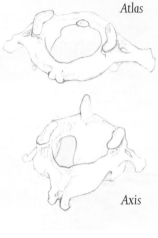

At the top of the cervical spine are two vertebrae known as atlas and axis. The axis inserts into the centre of the wide atlas bone above it. The upper diagram here shows the two bones separated, with the atlas on top. The diagram below shows how they fit together, with the upward-protrusion of the axis bone fitting through the atlas and so into the base of the skull, allowing the head to fit onto the neck vertebrae. This allows the head to be stable yet move freely.

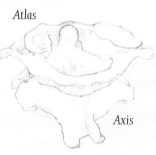

This needs a free-moving spine and strong deep back and neck muscles and ligaments. Crucially, the enormous lumbar vertebrae (the lower spine) need to support the much narrower and smaller neck vertebrae.

How the atlas sits on the axis

On the next page, study the drawing of the internal structure of the neck, how the passages from the mouth and nose go into the neck, how it's the job of the epiglottis to differentiate between food and air and so open appropriately. Remember how relatively rare it is to get that wrong and choke. Notice the nasal concha.

The name 'concha' has been borrowed from the conch shell, as the nasal passages are likened to the spiralling of

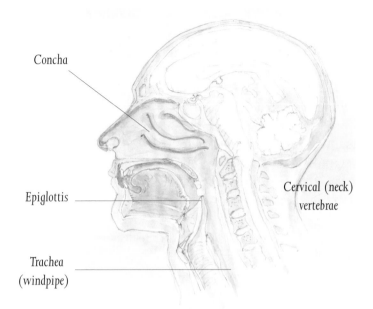

Concha

Epiglottis

Cervical (neck)
vertebrae

Trachea
(windpipe)

these shells. By this spiralling, the air coming in can be thoroughly warmed, cleansed and humidified, ready for the lungs. Amazingly the dust, pollution and infections are gathered up by the mucus and transported via the throat to the stomach, where the mix is sterilized by the stomach acid and eliminated. Hence the nasal concha is the first line of immunological defence in the body. This is particularly important during an epidemic.

In modern civilization, where we are so often supported by chairs, car seats and soft beds, the lumbar spine often does not have the strength, length and flexibility to give the lesser curve of the cervical vertebrae the support it needs for the heavy head. Thus, if the lumbar spine is curved back, the head tends to drop forward, and then we have to lift the head using the neck vertebrae and neck muscles, which inevitably puts a strain on the neck. In turn this makes the throat tighten up and the vocal diaphragm constrict. Thus it closes the air passages from the nose to the trachea – known as the windpipe. So then mouth breathing feels necessary.

If the feet and legs are not stood straight up through the pelvis to connect to the lumbar spine via the main hip flexor muscle, the psoas, then the lumbar spine collapses forward and down on the pelvis and we tend to push from the pelvis to propel ourselves forward. Again the chin has to lift forward and up, too much, to balance the heavy weight of the head. The top of the nasal passages are then constricted, so again mouth breathing feels necessary.

You can see the psoas muscle in the diagram below. It originates all the way from the twelfth thoracic vertebra and each lumbar vertebra down the lumbar spine and inserts on the top of the inner thigh bone (on the lesser trochanter of the femur

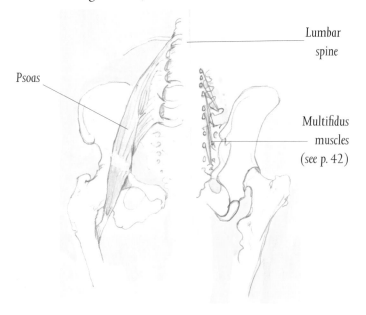

Lumbar
spine

Psoas

Multifidus
muscles
(see p. 42)

bone). This is the most important hip flexor muscle, and from the standing up of the long thigh bone into the hip socket, it allows the lumbar spine to lengthen up off the sacrum bone,which in turn lengthens the crura muscles (shown in the diagram on p. 40, and likened to the strings that hold a parachute up and insert down the front of the lumbar spine) down to move the diaphragm down and out (left side of diagram). Then on the right side of the diagram are the powerful deep back muscles that connect the sides of the vertebrae (the transverse processes) to one another to allow the spine to strengthen and elongate. Then the lumbar spine can lengthen up to its natural length and curve and so hold the whole upper body up off the pelvis. In order for the thigh bone to stand up into the hip socket, the feet need to be engaged into the ground, with the arch of the foot lifted and the ankle bones lifted off the downward movement of the heel.

To the right, the diagram of the lungs shows how the trachea (windpipe) divides into the left and right bronchus, about a third of the

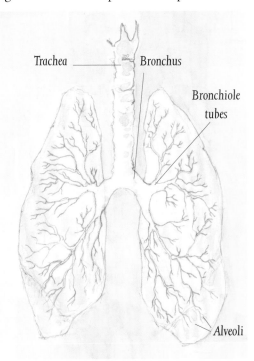

Trachea

Bronchus

Bronchiole tubes

Alveoli

way down the lungs. This is so the breath can go down, sideways, towards the back and top of the lungs relatively evenly. You can see that the lower part of the lungs is bigger and wider than the top so there are more alveoli (see below) at the bottom and back of the lungs. For this reason it is very important for the breath to be able to spread down. Breathing at a fast rate, using more the top, secondary respiratory muscles (the pectorals and the sternocleidomastoid muscles), does not make full use of the lower lung lobes,. As a result, the absorption of oxygen into the haemoglobin is not so efficient, reducing oxygenation of the blood and decreasing vitality.

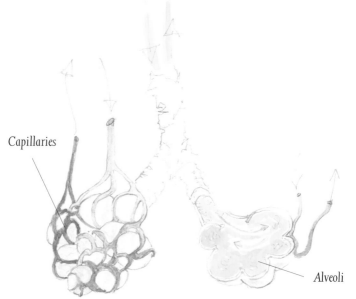

Capillaries

Alveoli

The Alveoli are the cauliflower-like clusters at the end of the bronchiole tubes that have many hundreds of fine capillaries gathered over them for the oxygen to diffuse into the reddish capillaries (fine blood vessels) and the carbon dioxide to diffuse into the rather bluer capillaries. On the right, a cross-section.

Abdominal Breathing (a practice to forget)

*'Do not inflate the abdomen while inhaling as this prevents
the lungs from expanding fully. Breathing in or out must be
neither forcible nor quick, for strain of the heart or
damage to the brain may result.'*

Sri B.K.S.Iyengar, LIGHT ON PRANAYAMA

*'Each of the yoga poses is accompanied by breathing and it
is during the process of exhalation that the spine can stretch
and elongate without effort. We learn to elongate and extend,
rather than pull push. Elongation and extension can only
occur when the pulling and pushing have come to an end.
This is the revolution.'*

Vanda Scaravelli, AWAKENING THE SPINE

When people want to breathe more, they often think this
means work with the abdomen. The abdomen does not
breathe, however; the abdomen is separated from the lungs by
the thoracic diaphragm. There is no direct connecting system
between them. I am amazed that the concept of 'abdominal
breathing' still persists in yoga teaching. I even heard it being
taught very recently on 'Woman's Hour' on BBC Radio 4.

We only feel the need to push and pull the abdomen in
breathing because the lumbar vertebrae are too collapsed
down on one another and too pushed forward and down on
the sacrum through bad posture. So it is thought that the abdomen needs to protrude to make space for the diaphragm
moving down. In fact, the thoracic diaphragm does not move
down very much – around one and a half centimetres (half an
inch) during natural breathing – not enough to displace the
abdominal organs in any significant way. It moves more out-
wards, taking the ribs with it. The movement is likened to the

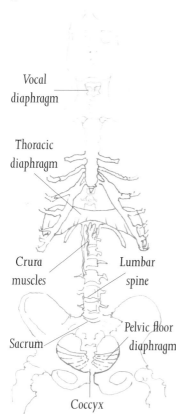

Vocal diaphragm

Thoracic diaphragm

Crura muscles

Lumbar spine

Sacrum

Pelvic floor diaphragm

Coccyx

undulations of a jellyfish.

In the hours of research for this book, I looked at many videos of all sorts of *pranayama* (breath awareness), practised mostly by twenty- to forty-year olds and did not see anyone at all who sat with an aligned, elongated and awakened spine! All were collapsed in the abdomen, and the shoulders were collapsed and hunched on the ribs, so breathing by pushing and pulling the abdomen felt necessary for these young people.

During lockdown, I have been having one-to-one Zoom sessions with a teacher in the Scaravelli tradition, Diane Long. They are the toughest, most demanding half hours of my present schedule! The instructions on sitting for *pranayama* are the hardest to maintain of any of the postures: sitting forward on the top of the thigh bones, with the coccyx travelling down out of the sacrum, the sacrum moving in and up, the shoulder blades moving into the ribs, the hands engaged into the ground! See the *asana* chapter, no. 3, for more detailed instruction. The photos opposite speak for themselves.

Let's explore how the spine moves with the breath, without abdominal pushing or inflating.

Lying down on the floor or outside on the earth and with the feet flat on the ground, bring your awareness down the

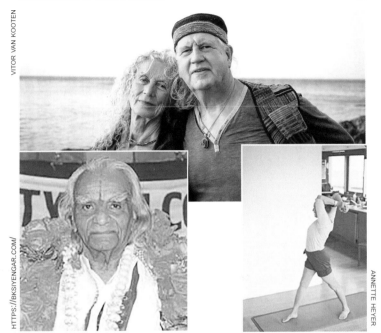

VITOR VAN KOOTEN

HTTPS://BKSIYENGAR.COM/

ANNETTE HEYER

Yoga teachers: Angela Farmer and Victor van Kooten in their eighties,
Sri B.K.S. Iyengar in his nineties and Diane Long in her seventies

length of your body to the base of the spine (the tailbone or
coccyx). Exhale without pushing the breath out, and wait for
the breath to come in of its own accord.

Observe what happens as you inhale. Can you feel how
the coccyx (tail bone) moves away from the flat sacrum bone
towards your heels? Notice what happens as you exhale. Does
the lengthening continue?

Inhaling again, as the coccyx moves away from the sacrum,
can you feel the lumbar vertebrae moving forward and upwards, off the sacrum towards the upper back, making a long,
gentle arch of the lumbar spine, through the midline of the
abdominal area – and then returning back only slightly as you

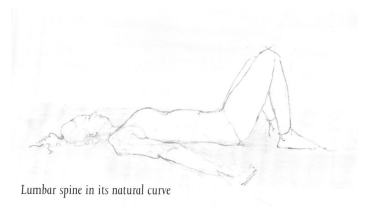

Lumbar spine in its natural curve

exhale? In this way, the lumbar spine can go on lengthening and strengthening as you go on focusing on your breathing.

You may find that with practice over time, the two-way lengthening of the spine increases. This in turn engages all the deepest back muscles, the multifidus (see p. 36). These are considered the most powerful muscles in the body.

Also, the intermediate back muscles and the layers of abdominal muscles all engage back towards the spine, toning and lengthening, with the inhalation. They maintain this length with the exhalation. So the whole abdominal area becomes like a smooth long natural corset, no pushing required! This of course then needs to be maintained as the natural posture – hence the need to practice *asana*.

It would also be useful to lie on your tummy – prone – to be aware of how your breathing changes. Put your arms up to your face so that your brow can rest on your hands. You can then feel that the breath comes more into the lower back of the lungs, because the ribs can move away from the spine more easily. You can also feel the very gentle, slight, natural movement of the abdomen – emphasizing that you do not need to push or pull at all.

In hospital, Covid-19 patients who have had great difficulty breathing are turned to lie prone for a short period to enable the breath to come in more deeply and easily. They are then turned at regular intervals from side to back to front.

You may like next to look at the instructions for sitting in Chapter 3, in the asanas (noting how Sophy Hoare is sitting here). Can you retain the length and engagement of the lumbar spine and all the layers of muscles around it as you sit to breathe? This takes much continued practice.

As you go on breathing, can you feel that the back ribs move slightly out of the upper back to make more space for the breath to come into the back of the lungs?

The Biochemistry of Breathing

A biochemist would say that the level of carbon dioxide in the blood is what instigates the inhalation. There is a great deal of debate about the interchange of oxygen and carbon dioxide. Once, it was considered that carbon dioxide was merely a waste gas that has to be eliminated from the lungs, and that we need to take in as much oxygen as we can – to the extent that pure oxygen is given when there are breathing problems. Current research is showing that there is a balance to be found between oxygen and carbon dioxide. We need carbon dioxide as much as we need oxygen.

A biophysicist would say the change of pressure in the lungs relative to outside the lungs instigates the inhalation. You can feel this change if you pause at the end of a full exhalation: the feeling of needing to expand the lungs, as the pressure from the outside of the ribs is exerted on the lungs. Then, at the top of the inhalation, there is naturally more pressure on the inside of the lungs, than outside, and this is what makes us exhale.

Both are true, however it has been recently found that car-

bon dioxide is the significator and key variable here, the one
that causes the change from the exhalation to the inhalation,
while the important pause at the end of the exhalation creates
a more balanced respiratory action.

The Balance of Oxygen and Carbon Dioxide

It has been commonly assumed that the carbon dioxide we
breathe out is simply a waste product. Quite the opposite is
true: we need carbon dioxide (CO_2) just as much as we need
oxygen. A simple balance is important. This has implications
for how we breathe out.

> 'In 1904 the Danish biochemist, Christian Bohr, discovered
> that carbon dioxide facilitates the release of oxygen to the
> cells. Oxygen is carried around the body in the haemoglobin,
> in the red blood cells. Bohr discovered that carbon dioxide
> acts as the catalyst for haemoglobin to release its load of oxy-
> gen for use by the body. When levels of carbon dioxide in the
> blood are low, the bond between oxygen and haemoglobin
> increases. This means that the body cannot access the oxygen
> in the blood and it leads to poor body oxygenation.

> 'In 2017, a doctor at Subharti Medical College in India,
> wrote a detailed review of the benefits of carbon dioxide. The
> paper's author, Dr Singh, is a yoga practitioner and has ded-
> icated much time to researching how yoga works. Dr Singh
> discovered that CO_2 stimulates the vagus nerve, an impor-
> tant cranial nerve…. He discovered that increased levels of
> CO_2 in the blood could activate the vagus nerve and slow the
> heart rate. He describes CO_2 as "natural sedative". It soothes
> the irritability of the brain's conscious centres promoting our
> ability to use logic, reason and common sense.

'Without CO_2 we can become anxious, depressed and angry.'
THE BREATHING CURE by Patrick Mckeown

Over-breathing

It is common to be given the instruction, 'Take a deep breath in and push the breath out' in many forms of exercise and even in yoga classes. This tends to be forceful and noisy, and actually creates what is called over-breathing – that is, taking in too much air too suddenly and too quickly and too much into the top of the chest. It disturbs the balance of oxygen and carbon dioxide because it tends to push out too much carbon dioxide – so you then have to force the breath in again.

Over-breathing, also called upper airway breathing is actually hyperventilation, and it can happen when we are anxious, frightened and stressed: when we feel that we cannot get our breath in properly, so we breathe in too much, too quickly into the top chest – and actually get too much oxygen in and exhale too much carbon dioxide from the lungs.

This happens in respiratory conditions such as asthma. In an asthma attack, there is a feeling of not being able to breathe, so actually this is a case in which over-breathing tends to happen. With someone during an asthma attack, I have asked them to bring the spine parallel to the ground, with the arms over a table or

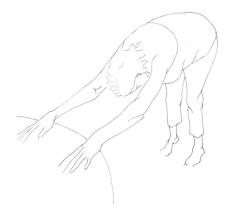

chair, and have put my hands on the lower rib asking them to feel the ribs move in and out as they breathe. This has made the attack subside. Of course, it may not happen in every case; the person I was with has always been a yoga practitioner and able to trust and be with and in their body and aware of their breath. Yet the position they were in brings the breath into the lower lungs and so calms the breathing and therefore the whole body, mind and person.

Jaw Dropping

There is also developing research in orthodontics, where it has been regular practice to take teeth out if it is deemed that they are too many for the mouth. The research shows that our mouths are actually getting smaller: too small for the number of teeth we are supposed to have. By contrast, indigenous people have been found to have wide arches to their mouths and straight teeth.

One area of the research has looked at Caribbean grandparents, who were eating natural unprocessed foods that needed a lot of chewing. The result was that they developed good musculature in the jaw. They came to live in England and their grandchildren ate mostly soft, processed food. Even over a couple of generations, those jaws were found to have dropped and their faces narrowed, and teeth had to be removed.

It can happen even more quickly. In further research, a young boy had a pet gerbil sleeping in his room without realizing that he was allergic to its fur. The congestion caused by the allergy made him unable to breathe through his nose. His orthodontist found that his whole jaw and tongue had dropped and narrowed to make space in his mouth for him to breathe totally through his mouth so the space for the teeth

was too narrow. Charles Eisenstein, in his book, THE YOGA OF
EATING, says,

> 'The unnatural eating habits that we impose on our body are
> similar in nature and origin to the unnatural patterns we im-
> pose on our breath. The breath in fact could be viewed as
> another form of eating, in which we take in a substance nec-
> essary for life and expel waste products for the environment
> to recycle.
>
> 'Just as we are hurried eaters, we are hurried breathers. Just
> as we have become numb to our bodies' authentic appetites
> for food, so we have also lost touch with the natural rhythms
> of our breath.
>
> 'Recovering naturalness in breathing is a practice and a tool
> for recovering naturalness in eating.'

In both areas – breathing and eating – we can gain sensitivity
to body messages and learn to trust those messages. Eating
mindfully to appreciate and enjoy our food, we need to slow
down – not be in a hurry!

I grew up with two brothers who were constantly hungry,
and one of them in particular would take food from my sister's
plate and mine, if they could – so we learned to eat fast! Often,
we try to do other things while eating, as though we do not
have time to eat. This plays havoc with our digestion.

In 2020, I had an extended retreat in a Theravada Buddhist
monastery. In my time there we were expected to eat slowly and
silently, giving the food our full attention, chewing each mouthful, not putting too much in the mouth at once, and finishing
one mouthful before taking another. We did not eat bits and
pieces, snacks or food from the table whilst cooking, or when
receiving the blessing from the monks and nuns, and we didn't
go for seconds. This is a traditional practice in India and other

Eastern countries, and it is a challenging and powerful way of addressing long-term habits in a society that can often simply 'eat on the run'. In France and Italy eating also has a more important place than in English-speaking countries, so more time is taken really to enjoy it – all afternoon or evening sometimes.

If you happen to have given up meat, there is plenty in a vegetarian diet to chew on. My favourites are walnuts straight out of their shells (fresher, and great for the brain), crisp apples, Brazil nuts, raw carrot, radish, fennel, lettuce – what else can you find that needs a lot of mastication?

Vegetarianism and veganism fit with the yogic principle of *ahimsa*, non-violence. Another yogic activity, Sanskrit chanting, when practised as originally taught with clear enunciation, gives much exercise to all the mouth and throat. It is a practice we will return to in chapter 6.

Gesture

Mudra, translated as gesture, is an important part of yoga practice. Some of them are *kaya mudra* body gestures. *Kaya mudra* are postures that are rested into for some time, such as *viparita karani mudra*, meaning reversing attitude gesture. We shall look at this posture in chapter 3. In *pranayama* meditation there are also hasta mudras, hand gestures that assist in focusing the heart and mind, such as *padma mudra,* the lotus gesture (see p. 92). *Khechari mudra*, a *kaya mudra* (see instructions for both of these in the *pranayama* chapter, no. 4) can help with the shape of the mouth. In *khechari mudra*, the tip of the tongue is placed on the roof of the mouth. It also feels that this broadens and lifts the roof of the mouth. The effect is increased when *brahmari* (humming bee) breath is sounded.

Interestingly, craniofacial experts are starting to recommend a practice akin to *khechari mudra*, often known as 'mewing', in which the tongue is similarly placed. One of the scientists, Professor Mike Mew, whose subject is craniofacial dystrophy, recommends that the tongue is placed firmly on the roof of the mouth, as it has such strong musculature that it would, in time, broaden and lift the roof of the mouth.* With the face, mouth and jaw, it is good to be aware that the fascia around and containing all the internal organs is malleable: it can reduce, expand, change shape. This in turn lets the lungs expand considerably, giving a greater capacity and so increasing the oxygenation process.

This increased capacity of the lungs also applies even if you have been breathing into the top chest for years. With daily practice, together with a concerted effort to breathe also through the nose, the lung size and capacity can increase and the nostrils open yet more.

Over many years, I have watched my Vedic chanting teacher, Sarah Waterfield, as well as her students, to see how the face can be transformed and toned, lifting and opening the cheekbones up and out, taking away any sagging jaw, so that the capacity and awareness of the mouth has increased dramatically – and have felt this in myself from a regular daily practice of chanting. This greater capacity and awarenesss of the mouth will also affect the capacity of the lungs.

This feels rather dramatic, yet you only need to look at opera singers, and generally all singers, to see how the mouth and chest develop with movement.

Katharina Schroth had scoliosis and was bedridden as a teenager in Germany. She worked out a method of curing herself, through looking in the mirror to see where the restrictions in her spine were – and then consciously breathing

*See www.movewellapp.com/mewing101:thebeginner'sguide

into the lungs under those areas in many different positions, including regularly manoeuvring herself around on a table for five years. In that time, she had breathed her spine straight by moving and increasing the size and capacity of her lungs and restructuring the fascia that connected to her spine. She could move normally and started teaching other sufferers of scoliosis. Later she created a clinic where many people came and were cured. She spent the next sixty years taking this method into hospitals in Germany.

Cold Water Swimming and the Breath

Swimming, especially in the sea, is a very good and natural complement to yoga *asana* and *pranayama* – posture and breathing practice. It can be vigorous or relaxed and restful with the different strokes followed by floating looking at the sky. This is like *savasana* on a floating surface and is very meditative.

Having encountered the Bluetits Chill Swimmers (groups of swimmers all over the UK who swim all year round in the sea, rivers and lakes), I started swimming in the sea in Aberporth, near where I live, in October 2020 and continued into November. I started going again in February 2021. It is very stimulating on breathing and so energizing. Many claims are made about it now. I have always loved swimming in the sea and would go in whenever I can but have not disciplined myself to go in such cold water before.*

*Three online articles may be of interest: https://www. netdoctor.co.uk/healthy-living/fitness/a30499541/cold-water-swimming/ – then https://www.ncbi.nlm.nih.gov/pmc/articles/ PMC6334714 – and https://www.runnersworld.com/uk/news/ a34436175/can-cold-water-swimming-ward-off-dementia/

It certainly feels wonderful when you get used to it and wonderful afterwards, provided you get warm quickly and have a flask of hot drink ready for when you come out. I now hope to continue it all year.

When you first go in, the breath catches with the shock of the cold water – so you tend to hold your breath. If you pause at that point and regulate your breathing until it feels how you normally breathe, it will then be much easier to go into the cold water. Then as you move and swim, continue to be aware of your breathing. This will enable you to stay in and adjust to the temperature.

There is much research now being conducted on cold water swimming, especially on the hope that it may hold back the onset of dementia. As is often the case, the research is inconclusive as yet. Wim Hof, a pioneer, explains how it regulates the heart and so can reduce high blood pressure. I would feel that it depends how you breathe, day to day: it's essential to be aware of how the cold water affects your breathing. Your response will be very powerful gasps at the outset, especially when you first go in, and most particularly if you do not have a regular breathing practice that enables you to meet very cold water while maintaining an awareness of regular breathing. So I would highly recommend that you get breathing before you start!

Chapter 3 : Posture

'There is a division in the back where the spine moves simultaneously in two opposite directions: from the waist downwards towards the feet, which are pulled by gravity, and from the waist upwards, through the top of the head, lifting us up freely. The pull of gravity makes it possible for us to extend the upper part of the spine, and this extension allows us to also release tension between the vertebrae.
'This is a natural process, ever present in all upright living things, in trees, in growing flowers and in plants. The deeper the roots penetrate into the ground, travelling below the surface of the earth, the taller and stronger grows the tree.'

Vanda Scaravelli, AWAKENING THE SPINE

'Studies confirm that the two main pillars that support effective yoga practice are slow breath and attention"

Olga Kabel

Yoga and Breathing

Your posture – that is, how you stand, sit and walk and how you hold your body in whatever exercise you do – is, as the previous chapter demonstrates, intrinsically connected to how you breathe. We use the term 'full height' to describe our natural upright posture without any bending or sagging. Can you feel that if you stand up to your 'full height', without stiffening, it is much easier to breathe? You may find that the ribs can open more, and that the diaphragm can move, so the lungs can fill properly.

Traditionally, in the practice of yoga, *asana* (posture) is practised for some time – even for years – before we are ready to practise *pranayama* (breath awareness) in detail, because breathing is so tied up with feelings and habits, and the asanas are ways of letting these go. Here, I have attempted to give more natural ways of practising *pranayama* without years of asanas. However, it is still much better and easier if you have a regular practice of *asana* before practising *pranayama*. At the end of this book, I have suggested where you can find recommended teachers. Also you could look at two of my previous books, YOUR YOGA BODYMAP and STANDING, SITTING, WALKING, RUNNING. It also depends on the translation of *pranayama*, which does not mean how your control the breath but how you feel the life energy within.*

In fact, all yoga postures have the potential to change unhelpful breathing patterns. It does depend on how you do them, though! There is the gym habit of pushing and pulling the body – which has been adopted in some yoga teaching – forcefully imposing the mind on the natural intelligence of the body. Usually in the gym version this would be accompanied by holding the breath, forcing the breath in and out through the mouth as well as the nose.

Asana is one of the 'Eight Limbs' of yoga. The first two are the yamas and the niyamas, the 'Virtues', which are concerned with how you live your life in the world. Possibly the most important of these is *ahimsa*: non-violence in each and every aspect of your life, and very much including your yoga practice!

*For clarification of this point, see Alastair Shearer's explanation, quoted on p. 81

We can very subtly or forcefully push ourselves, thinking 'this will be doing us good' or we can beat ourselves up out of unconscious guilt. To work like this would be accompanied by a forceful inhalation, and often then a holding of the breath while in the posture. If we push ourselves hard, even in yoga, we are likely to cause an injury. So you need to be very aware of your body, in your practice and afterwards. If you have pain that continues after your practice, you most likely pushed yourself – probably in the area that hurts. If you give your full attention to what you are doing, moment by moment, and how you are breathing, this will not happen.

There is what I call good pain and there is what I call bad pain! Many students, I have found, find this distinction amusing; they have a laugh about it. That's fine, as it makes them relax! Good pain is moving an area of the body – the spine, a muscle, a joint, a tendon, fascia – that has not been moved in that way for a while, so that you become more aware of it. Some of us would call that pain, but it is more of a waking up. If it subsides when you come out of that posture, then it is indeed a waking up.

If it persists, then it is bad pain, and you have pushed yourself unhelpfully in that area.

It is also common for areas of the body to be under strain and in pain because another area of the body is not doing its job properly. If we can find that area and wake it up, this will take the strain off the painful area.

The concept of 'waking up' is important in this book, so I will explain it further. As an example, most people are not aware of their feet, which are far too far from their heads! If the inner ankles pronate – that is, roll down and in, which is very common when the arch of the foot is not employed to lift them up – then the hips and lumbar spine will collapse down on the thigh bones, and the knees will have to brace back to take the weight of this collapse down. Thus, bringing our awareness to the lift of the arch and the lift of the ankle bones away from the heel, and standing much more on the outside of the feet, will eventually take strain off the knees, hips and lower back.

This takes constant awareness – hence the expression 'waking up' – and it will make the feet ache for a while. As you can imagine, this is what I term good pain. The same thing can be achieved by taking the weight more forward and onto ball of the foot and toes. The expression 'on the ball' is literal – it's how toddlers first walk. Then, keeping the lift of the ankle bone which that forward move gives, the heel can then go down without heaviness rather than 'digging the heels in', another literal expression – for obstinacy.

Moving the weight forward has the effect of lifting the long thigh bone more up into the hip socket, which in turn gives the lift of the lumbar spine off the pelvis and thus the lift, too, of the upper body off the knees and pelvis.

One of the highest causes for absences from work is lower back pain. Generally the remedy, unless there is structural damage, is to wake up the feet and their connection to the legs! However this needs constant awareness of how we move and practice over time, but I have experienced it working for myself and many of my students and other yoga practitioners.

This philosophy of developing awareness, being awake to our bodies, is central to our awakening to good breathing habits. If we think back to Vanda Scaravelli's remarks at the beginning of this chapter, the spine in the western body tends to be trapped between tight hips and strained shoulders. So by focusing on moving the spine and freeing the shoulders and hips, the whole body will be released from strain and will 'wake up'! The feet and legs can then connect up through the pelvis to the spine. This is the basic principle of Vanda Scaravelli's teaching and of Scaravelli-inspired yoga.

This way of practice is very specific and it is necessary to have a teacher who understands it. We tend to stay in old habits if we are too long on our own in any practice. However, you are encouraged and expected to do your own practice in between classes. I have given some useful teacher links at the end of the book.

If the postures are practised yogically – that is, without pushing or straining but with your full attention and focus, your breath moving with the movement of the body and vice versa (without trying to make it do so) – you will find it quite hard work. Indeed, you need to find it hard work as it moves the body in a different way from the 'push–pull' method. It is also aerobic if practised in this deep, thorough way, with the mind giving the body its full and undivided attention. Music plugged into the ears is a distraction!

Breath Awareness

It would be good also to take time to observe, without influencing the outcome, which comes first: the breath moving the body or the body moving the breath?

There is a tendency when we are so 'up in our heads', as most of us are today, for the head to lead and drag the body behind it in both our practice and life! This in itself tends to make us hold our breath. If the movement and the breath can come together more from the intelligence of the body, then the head is kept stable, moving with the body rather than leading. This regulates the breath and ensures that we are breathing through the nose.

This applies to all postures, but the postures recommended below are ones in which you can pause and become aware of how the breath is in the body.

The postures are best moved into on an exhalation (except for *bhujangasana* – serpent or cobra pose). However, trying to make this happen can become too mechanical if the practice is forceful. For the first few years simply be aware that you are breathing and the practice of the postures themselves will change how you breathe.

The yoga teacher most responsible for bringing the practice of *asana* to the Western world, Sri B. K. S. Iyengar, has said that we are beginners for the first twenty years of yoga practice! I was taught by Mr Iyengar that the practice of the postures must come first to move the spine, diaphragm and shoulders and change the way we stand, walk and move, so that the breath comes in and out easily and is more ready for *pranayama* – awareness of breathing.

Mr Iyengar would often emphasise that *pranayama* is more difficult to practise than the *asanas* or postures. I have found that certainly to be true, and there is also some resistance in people to notice how they breathe at all, because it is linked to the feelings. Maybe also we have a tendency to expect cures to be effected for us from the outside, without us having to do anything at all. This book is designed to show that the whole process is much more natural than generally thought.

We will now move on to some recommended postures to start this process so it gradually becomes a habit, thus increasing lung capacity.

The Postures

Tadasana with hands on the wall or a broad trunk of a tree

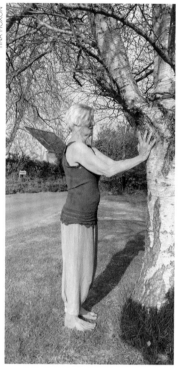

Tadasana means 'as it is now'. However, the pose often is called mountain pose. At the end of this chapter you will find another pose, *parvatasana*, which is the one that actually means 'mountain'.

Stand facing a tree or a wall, which should be about the length of your arms away from you. Put your hands on it at shoulder height with your elbows relaxed down, but with your hands and arms fully engaged into the wall or tree so that you are working hard to engage the upper arm into the shoulder socket.

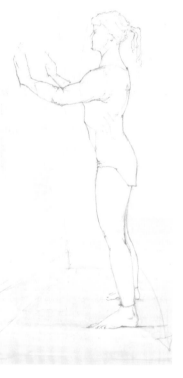

Feel the connection from the fingertips, through the hands, arms and shoulder socket to your scapula (shoulderblades) to bring them in towards the ribs, away from your spine and slightly down your back.

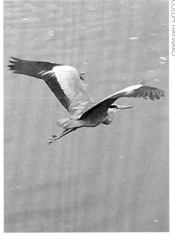

Stand your feet firmly down into the ground, your ankle-bones lifting off the heel bone. The thighbones then stand straight up into the hips, and the lumbar spine engages up off the pelvis, helping you breathe easily and naturally. When you feel all of that, let the arms fly up and out as though you have an air current underneath them like a bird's wing.

Tadasana with wall or tree behind you

Now turn around, away from the tree or wall, and stand about your own foot's distance from it (or a shorter distance if you have a tendency to push your lumbar spine forward and so strain your back or sacrum).

Spread forward onto the balls of your feet and spread out through your toes, lengthening up through the front thighs so as to take the pubic bone back towards the sacrum. This will lengthen the spine forward and up, in the direction of the top of the spine, and ease the head up off the neck vertebrae. The shoulders broaden and arms fly up like a bird again. Bring the fingertips over your head to lightly touch the wall or tree, ease them into it without pushing, so that the shoulders broaden and the upper spine can move through the shoulders.

Keep the fingers lightly on the wall and stand the feet, espe-

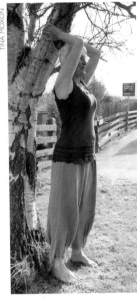

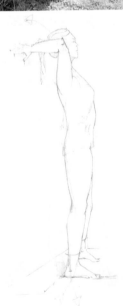

cially the heels, down into the ground to bring the sacrum bone in and up. Lengthen the lumbar spine and cervical vertebrae forward and up, feeling the spread and roundness of the back of the head to give the impetus to bring the arms over and down.

Now you are standing free of the wall or tree in *tadasana*, having 'brought yourself up to your full height' by the last two postures. Can you feel how you are breathing now? Here are some questions to ask yourself:

• When your breath comes in, do your feet engage more with the ground underneath you, especially if you are outside? – as though you are a tree sending your roots into the earth in order for your trunk (spine) to grow up towards the sky and your branches (limbs) to open out.

• Or does it happen the other way around for you? That is, that the awareness of the contact that your feet make with the ground encourages your breath to come in? How amazing our bodies are!

• What happens to the contact of your feet to the ground when your breath goes out?

• Does the roundness of your

heels find more contact with the ground?

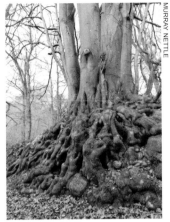

Note the extraordinary connection a tree has with the earth.

Padangustasana, one leg lifted

Stand in *tadasana*, as you have just done. Stand firmly up through one leg, by spreading the foot into the ground and lengthening up from the ankle bone through the thighbone

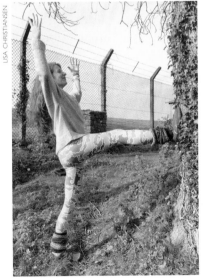

into the hip socket. Then, bend the other leg up so that the knee joint comes above the hip joint. Put the foot on a chair or a ledge, or against a wall or tree, as Tina is doing in the photograph.

Can you be aware that this posture naturally brings the breathe more into the back of the lungs by spreading the back ribs away from the spine?

Tadasana with hand on the wall or tree to open side ribs

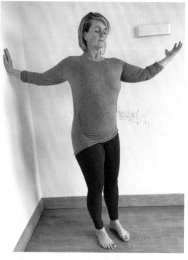

Start with both hands on the wall, as in the drawing on p. 60, and then, turn your feet away from the wall and bring the hand off the wall as Lisa is doing in the picture. Let your arm open out to the side like an Indian dance movement. Spread firmly down through the balls of your feet and out through your toes as though you are spreading them like the roots in the picture, into the ground.

Can you feel how that movement opens the side ribs and the whole shoulder girdle, so increasing the opening of the ribs away from the spine? As a result, the breath then spreads more deeply into the lungs, increasing the lung capacity.

Then feel the movement down through the heels which gives the movement forward and up of the spine through the shoulders to the crown. Turn your feet to put both hands back on the wall and go to repeat this on the other side.

Then if you could find two

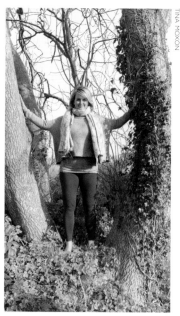

TINA MOXON

trees, or a double-trunked one, as Lisa has in the second photo, you could put a hand on each trunk to feel the movement
into both sides of the ribs and the opening in the armpit to let
the lymph flow more easily from the nodes there. How does
that effect the movement of the breath through the body?

If there is no suitable tree handy, then – spreading the arms
to the side – ease the heel of the hand away as though you
wanted to take the walls away from one another to give a similar effect. Now you are ready and prepared for:

Vrksasana, Tree Pose

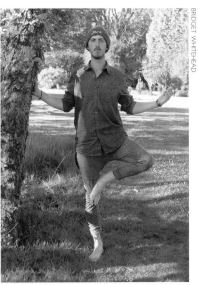

In the picture, Jared is using his hand on the tree
in *vrksasana*, tree pose, to
keep the standing leg in
and up like the trunk of a
tall, straight tree.

Begin by putting both
hands on the tree or wall
at shoulder height – facing
it, as on p. 60. Then turn
your feet at right angles
to the tree, as here, and
stand firmly down into the
Earth, through your foot
that's nearest the tree. In
this leg, lift the ankle bones up off the heel bone, gather the
thigh bone in and up into the hip socket.

Then lift the other heel and arch the foot so that you spring
off the ball of the foot, lifting the knee high up above the
hip. Bring the foot into the thigh of the standing leg. From
the firmness of the heel going down into the ground, stand

up through the spine, so that the chest, lungs and heart area spread out from the back ribs into the side ribs and the front ribs move away from the sternum. Maybe the arms will naturally move up and out like a wide spreading oak tree. To come out of the pose, lift the knee high above the hip, and then bring the leg forward to bring it down, as it is important to come out of any posture the way you went into it.

Turn around to do the same other side.

Using Peripheral Vision in a Standing Posture

As you perform these standing postures, one thing your developing awareness may cause you to notice is that there are subtle differences in your vision as you go into them stage by stage. What follows is something a colleague wrote to explore the difference in concentric vision and peripheral vision, and especially to see how that affects our breathing. She acknowledges two sources, but it is all in her own words.

'Back in 2012, the BBC programme 'Country File' featured a bushcraft type of person. He was talking about when we lived more with nature, and he was explaining about peripheral vision. He told us how we had tended to lose the ability to be able to be more in our peripheral vision, and how useful it was to retain this if you were wanting to really connect with your surroundings. He gave us a technique to help re-establish peripheral vision.

'This was to stand (preferably outside) and bring the hands together in front of you at the level of your breastbone, and then start to take the arms out wide to the sides, keeping the hands in sight all the time. This is your peripheral vision. After you have practised this over time, it always feels very relaxing on the brain, the mind and the thoughts, and restful for the eyes.

'In a later episode, the programme went on to consider predator vision and prey vision and how they are different. The predator has its eyes further forward on the head and the prey has its eyes more to the side of the head. This is so that the predator can hone in on its prey, while the prey can have an almost 360-degree

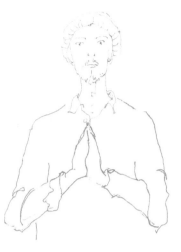

vision to see where an attack may be coming from. It seems that humans have a bit of both.

'Dona Holleman wrote a book called DANCING THE FLAME OF LIFE* in which she talks about predator and prey vision, relating them to yoga. I was excited to hear what she had to say – it brought together what I had been practising over the last few months. You may like to give this a go.

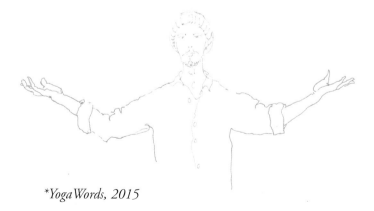

*Yoga Words, 2015

'When in predator vision, which is also called concentric view, you look through the corners of the eyes and you really focus in on an object – the object is very clear and three-dimensional and everything around it is a little blurred. When you are in prey or peripheral vision, you expand your vision out to 180 degrees. The field of vision softens and you become much more aware when something pops into your field of vision.

'This may also give an awareness of what is going on in the brain. Concentric (predator) vision is connected to the 'new' brain, the cerebrum, which is the linguistic brain, the brain that computes, analyses, fragments – the thinking brain. The prey vision or peripheral vision is connected to the 'old' reptilian brain or cerebellum. This is very much to do with our instinctual nature, before language, and with the fight-or-flight response.

'In concentric vision the internal dialogue is very easy, but in peripheral vision it is not. The two are mutually exclusive. Have a go for yourself. Look at an object and notice where you see it from, then think a few thoughts to yourself, and again notice where you are seeing from. Then go to peripheral vision. You will not be able to think inside your head, as if you do you will notice you start to look back through the corners of the eyes.

'So it is helpful to be able to access both. In yoga, for instance, with concentric vision we can look at a body piece by piece: see what the shoulder is doing, the foot, the ribs, etc; but in peripheral vision we can access the feeling of what is happening, the energy: we can see the whole.

'In her book Dona goes on to expand this to hearing. We can have concentric hearing and we can have peripheral hearing. In concentric hearing we hone in on a sound. When we do this it will usually have a reaction attached to it, For instance, a bird sound is a nice sound, but a car sound is not. When we are absorbed in these judgments we are not really hearing the sounds. If we can expand out into peripheral hearing, then the field of hearing becomes silence; and in that silence sounds pop up, received in the body as a vibration of air. There is no judgment attached. The only reaction on the body is how loud the sound is – not because it is a nice or not nice sound. Again, we can access both, the practice is knowing when to listen to both, so we can enjoy language and thinking and silence and feeling the totality of life.'

Bridget Whitehead

Exploring Peripheral Vision and its Connection to Breathing

As you use the instructions given by Bridget for exploring peripheral vision, notice how your breath is moving in and moving out. Notice when your hands are together over your breastbone in *namaste* and notice what movement there is in your body as the breath comes in and goes out.

Then when you extend the arms to the side, keeping your fingertips in your line of vision, pause, and feel again how your breath is moving in and out and what movement there is in your body as you breathe in and out.

Is there more movement in the top of your chest across the collarbones and top of the shoulderblades with the hands together in namaste, and when you are engaging more concentric vision? Is there more movement in the thoracic diaphragm, and do the lower back and side ribs open more when you take the arms out to the side and engage peripheral vision?

Would this simple movement help you engage the primary respiratory muscles – that is, the thoracic diaphragm, the intercostal muscles that are between the ribs, and the long abdominal rectus muscle that originates at the bottom of the xiphisternum and inserts on the top of the pubic bone so engaging it back to the lumbar spine – rather than the secondary respiratory muscles such as the pectorals at the top of the lungs?

More Helpful Postures for Breathing

Balasana, cat pose

Come down onto all fours with the hands directly underneath the shoulders and the knees directly underneath the hips. Imagine and feel what a cat looks like when it stands like this – or, better still, look at a cat when it wants to jump up onto a wall or when it is angry (as in the inset picture): how it arches its back up first. Can you do this by gathering up through your limbs to connect to the spine?

Can you do it so that the thoracic spine stands up and the back ribs then can move away from the spine, bringing the breath into the back of the lungs, as in the drawing below?

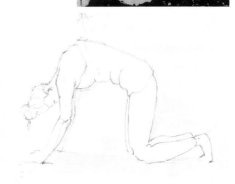

WOODCUT BY MURRAY NETTLE

Sixty per cent of lung capacity is at the back of the ribs, but we do not tend to use them enough. So feel the full expansion of the lungs here to take the breath

deep into the
alveoli – the
air sacs – where
the oxygen dif-
fuses into the
blood and the
carbon dioxide
diffuses out of
the blood (see
the diagrams in

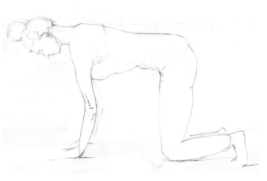

the anatomy chapter, pp. 36, 38).

Relax the back down as you exhale but do not push the lumbar forward and down as is often done in cat pose. Rather, pause and feel the effect of that full inhalation into the back. This is a cat ready to go for a stalk – with the head and ears alert (see the drawing above). These two movements create an opening of the ribs and awareness of how the breath then moves more into the lower back lungs.

Pindasana, embryo pose
Now relax the hips back onto the heels and let the head relax to the ground (if this is uncomfortable for you, sit on a chair leaning forward.).

Both the cat and the embryo poses relax the spine into its

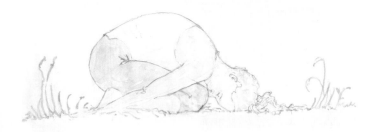

primary curve. This is the single curve that you were in, in the
womb. Again, allow the back ribs to spread and open away
from the spine with the inhalation, and the front of the body
to soften and relax back towards the back of the body with the
exhalation.

Setubandha sarvangasana, bridge pose
Now lie on your back with your feet firmly on the ground and
the knees bent, the kneecaps facing straight up towards the
ceiling. Become aware of your breathing. Feel the firmness of
your feet engaging into the earth. Bring your breath in, and as
you breathe out feel the length up through the legs to connect
through your pelvis to the spine, to move it forward and up
towards your head. Is the breath now wanting to go out? You
will feel that the upper back arches forward and up more easily, after being curved forward in the last two postures.

The arms can be spread to the side so that the side ribs and
armpits also open, allowing the lymph to move freely through
the body. Keep your head and throat relaxed and passive, your
eyes rested back.

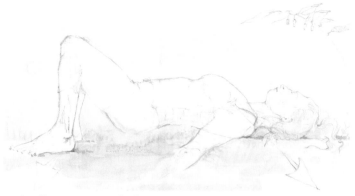

Setubandha sarvangasana, bridge pose

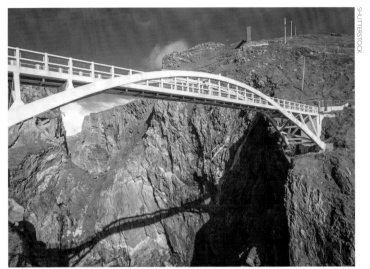

SHUTTERSTOCK

Mizen Head Bridge, Ireland; notice the way it is supported, just as the feet and the back of the skull support the movement of the spine forward and up

You can stay there for a few breaths, or put a support under your sacrum and rest there for five or ten minutes, aware of how the posture brings your breath in and out more slowly and deeply.

Viparita karani, waterfall

There are many ways to do these poses. After the practice of bridge pose, the spine is more flexible and the ribs more open, so that you can breathe more easily. The best way to begin is to put your legs up a wall, or a tree trunk if outdoors, with your hips just an inch or two away from the wall. In the picture overleaf, we are outdoors and using a tree. You can then feel the length of the coccyx (tailbone) down and away towards the wall and openness of the ribs, into the ground, to the side and to the front – all of which naturally brings the breath more deeply into the lungs. This is *viparita karani*, which means re-

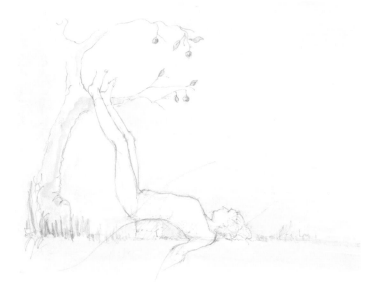

versing attitudes. It is sometimes called waterfall posture.

If you rest there for ten or
fifteen minutes it would gradually reverse an unhelpful attitude, over a time of regular
practice. Maybe it reminds
you of a waterfall?

If, after a while of practice,
you wish to go further, put
your feet onto the wall, firmly
engaging the feet into the wall
to take the spine forward and
up and the pelvis with it. Do
not push the pelvis or the sacrum – this is important.

Rest there and breathe for

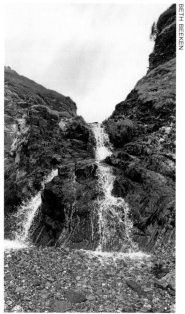

BETH BEEKEN

as long as it is comfortable and you can keep lifted, or put the support of a block or folded blanket underneath your pelvis to make the waterfall shape (as in the drawing on the previous page). Then feel how the ribs are even more open to give ease of breathing.

Do not go on to shoulderstand if you feel strained getting into it – go on to the next posture, staff pose. Shoulderstand will get easier as you practise all the other postures.

Salamba sarvangasana, shoulderstand

From *viparita karani*, turn around so that your head is three to six inches from the wall, your feet firm on the ground near your buttock bones, and then go into bridge pose again. As you come down from bridge pose, take your legs up and over your

head so that your toes tuck under, onto the wall (see the drawing). Go as high as you can, up onto the wall behind you. Keep your arms and hands firmly spread down on the ground be-hind you, so that your hips and up-per back lift for-ward and up.

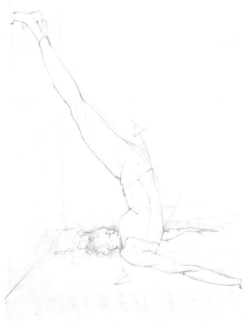

There is a ten-dency to put your hands on your

back to stay there but that makes the back slump back and
down onto the hands. You may not be able to stay long, but
the waking up of the deep, intermediate and surface back
muscles will enable you to breathe from the diaphragm right
down into the lower back lungs.

As you come slowly down, can you keep your head on the
ground? This is very important for the engagement of all the
diaphragms – throat (vocal), thoracic and pelvic floor – and so
that the abdomen does not grip and tighten. The diaphragms
can go into spasm from shock, trauma and coughing, and in-
verting them can release the spasm.

If it's difficult to stay there for a few minutes, relax the back
and hips on the ground with your legs lifted at a right angle to
your back as given in the next posture.

What do you notice about your breathing in this position?

Urdhva-mukha-dandasana, face-up staff pose

After bridge, and if you are leaving out shoulderstand, then
– lying on your back with your feet flat on the ground as for
bridge – lift your heels and spring off the ball of your foot.
This spring wakes up the arches of your feet – the plantar fascia, which makes the arch – which is essentially a diaphragm,
and thus connects to the thoracic and pelvic floor diaphragms
that move as you breathe. Hence the arches of the feet support
breathing from the diaphragms.

Let the spring of the feet off the toes lift the legs, to bring
them at right angles to the spine on the ground, spreading
the feet as though they were holding up the ceiling or sky so
that the legs lengthen to support and lengthen the spine (see
diagram on the next page).

Feel the spread of the back ribs on the ground away from the
spine as you breathe in and the slight rest back as you breathe

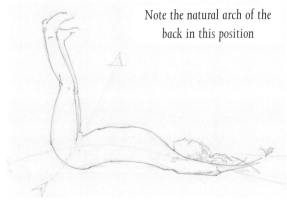

Note the natural arch of the back in this position

out. This does help the movement of the thoracic diaphragm. Do not grip and tighten the abdominal muscles to stay there, as this will tend to make you hold your breath. Stay there by lengthening up through the legs, and then gather the head of the long thighbone into the hip socket to bring the long abdominal rectus muscle back to the spine. Kofi Busia, a well-known advanced Iyengar teacher (now in teaching in Santa Cruz, California) used to make us stay there for twenty minutes! I now know why, after many years of practice: it really does wake up the legs and feet to connect to the spine, and so engages and tones all the layers of abdominal muscles back to the spine.

However, come down whenever you feel it's enough – but it is good to stay just a little longer after that feeling.

The springiness of the feet is very important in waking up the arch of the foot. I went – before all the lockdowns of 2020/21 – with my daughter to a running shop in Clapham. My daughter strides fast along the London pavements. Being much more used to the ups and downs of the cliff paths of west Wales, I have to run to keep up with her. So arrived with very sore feet in unsuitable sandals and felt I just had to try some trainers on!

To my amazement the assistants were saying that they now recommend flat soles, rather than all the support of the arches, as it makes your feet work more. I had felt this was so ever since I saw the strong supports given in trainers. Waking up the feet can transform them and even lift fallen arches with practice and perseverance. You do need to get professional advice, though, in case you have a medical need for support.

Of course I just had to buy some, if only to be able to walk back to South Norwood. They do make my feet work very hard and ache at first as I have to walk more on the outside of my feet specifically the outer two toes and the bones in the feet that connect to them. Yet they have done wonders for my feet, walking and yoga practice!

Jathara parivatanasana, lying twist of the spine

After shoulderstand and/or inverted staff pose, bring your feet onto the ground close to your hips. Lift your heels and hop your hips a few inches or centimetres to your right, so that your knees go over onto the ground to your left. Then you are over on the side of your left hip, keeping your toes active so that the engagement of your right toe into the ground lengthens up through the right thigh, into your hip, and relaxes your right shoulderblade to the ground.

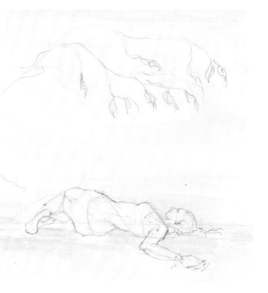

Focus on your breathing. In this position can you feel that the right ribs open out to the side, so that it seems easier to fill the right lung lobes? Relax into that breathing for several breaths, then use your toes, engaging into the ground to come back to the centre bring the hips central. Note how your breathing is now – and then go to the other side to repeat, in order that the left lung lobes increase their capacity to fill and empty, so increasing the oxygenation process.

It is helpful to repeat this as on the second time there is more movement through the spine and the ribs.

Rest with the feet down or the legs inverted up to bring you a symmetrical pose before coming up to sitting.

Sitting Postures

Parvatasana, mountain
Sit cross-legged on the ground or on an upright chair, with the outer edge of the feet engaged down into the ground along

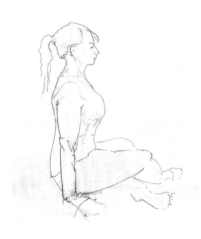

to the little toe. From that engagement down, the thighbones can gather back into the hip socket, so that the pubic bone and coccyx (tailbone) can engage down into the ground – with the result that you are sitting forward and up – on the top of the thigh bones, not back on the buttock bones. This brings the sacrum bone strongly in and up, lengthening the lumbar spine forward and up – so that the thoracic spine, ribs and lungs sit on the fulcrum of the first lumbar vertebra.

Take the whole of the hands strongly and firmly down into the ground or the side of the chair, gathering up from the elbows, bending the elbows back slightly, so that the upper arm gathers into its socket. The shoulderblades can then move slightly down and strongly into the ribs. This broadens the ribs, collarbone and shoulders, so lifting the shoulder girdle up off the ribs. The cervical spine then lengthens and comes into its natural curve, bringing the head directly up on the atlas bone, so the crown is in line with the coccyx..

This is very hard work and cannot be maintained for a long while without constant awareness – so when it is enough, lie down.

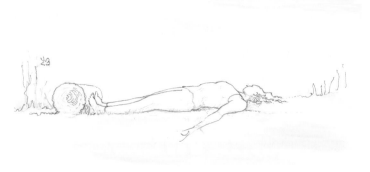

Savasana, relaxation
Now lie and relax in *savasana* – relaxation pose – head and eyes rested down, so that you can focus on your breath moving through your body for five or ten minutes.

Then you will be ready for any of the practices that follow in *pranayama* and chanting.

Yoga Nidra

I'm going to turn to another of my colleagues, Cryn Horn, for a few words about *yoga nidra.*

'It is generally understood that *yoga nidra* means 'yogic sleep'. Not "curled up under the duvet" kind of sleep, but more like the liminal place between deep dreamless sleep and being awake. A place where dreams often manifest.

'My understanding is that *yoga nidra* is a natural state, much as breathing is a natural state. The practices of *pranayama* can adapt the breath to achieve certain effects, but they all have to start with how a person is accustomed to breathe, however that is. Likewise, the practice of *yoga nidra* can be adjusted by the facilitator for different effects, but at its basic level it is a place where people very often go, quite naturally, when gazing at the sea, or into a garden, or at a loved one's face, or while washing up, or fishing, etc. Children access that place and are accused of daydreaming. It is a place where ideas can rise to the surface, problems get solved, and the body can reset its emotional, physical and energetic (pranic) states, allowing for profound rest and healing.

'Here in the West it is generally practised by listening to a facilitator, preferably live, but otherwise through a recording. The one who practises gets comfortable and suitably warm and follows the instructions. These usually start with settling the body, noticing how the body breathes, and then systematically observing what can be sensed with each of the major senses.

After that there might be a rotation of awareness around the body, some counting and/or visualization, and then a return to a more aware, alert state. Some schools insert a *sankalpa*, or intention, at the start and finish. You may or may not be consciously conscious through it all. The deeper mind can pay attention while the conscious mind can wander or switch off. Either is fine. If you have ever been in conversation with someone and you or the other person has said, 'Sorry, I missed that, I was miles away' then you have already experienced something similar to this practice.

'How each person reacts to *yoga nidra* tends to relate to what they need – so by listening to the same *yoga nidra* different people might get energy, relaxation, the solution to a problem, mental or physical healing, the ability to sleep, or just feeling better than they were at the start of the practice. (Or the same person listening to a specific *yoga nidra* on different days.)

'There have been attempts to trademark the state of *yoga nidra*, which is curious as it is a natural state, and has been observed by mystics the world over for thousands of years. The term *yoga nidra* may have come from India, but the practice is universal. If you would like to know more about this deep and nourishing practice then the Yoga Nidra Network is a good place to start. The founders, Uma Dinsmore-Tuli and Nirlipta Tuli, train facilitators in methods from a wide range of traditions. On the website there are many free Yoga Nidras available in a variety of languages, and an ever-expanding list of teachers.'*

*www.yoganidranetwork.org

Chapter 4 : Natural *Pranayama*

'The Sanskrit prānāyāma is usually taken to mean control (Yama) of the breath (prāna). Actually this is a misunderstanding. If we parse prānāyāma correctly, we get prāna and ayāma (the short last "a" of prāna and the short first "a" of ayāma elide by the rules of Sanskrit grammar to form one long ā.

'Strictly speaking prāna – cognate with the Greek pneuma and the Chinese chi – does not just mean "breath" but the cosmic life- energy that manifests on the gross level as breath in living creatures.

'Ayāma means "expansion, increase".

'Thus prānāyāma comes to mean "expansion and increase of life-energy." In other words, it is the process whereby the ordinary and relatively weak manifestation of prāna in the nervous system is purified and strengthened. Breathing exercises form part of this process, allowing the refined prāna to penetrate deeper into the nerves (nādis) of both gross and subtle anatomies and release blocks of accumulated stress,which in yogic terms is the whole contact of held and unresolved past experience-trapped memories,emotions, desires.

'As the nervous system becomes pure, this vitalizing flow of energy in the gross and subtle bodies increases....

'Breath and thought are two complementary expressions of prana; they go together. When the breath is calm, the mind automatically becomes more settled. One of the meanings of nirvana is "without breath".'

Alistair Shearer's Introduction
to THE YOGA SUTRAS OF PATANJALI

AWARENESS of how you breathe is the first step in your breath becoming more natural, and that awareness in itself will expand and increase the life energy, as it will alter how you breathe until it becomes a more regular, easier rhythm. So *pranayama* is not about a routine of practice that you do automatically – the mind dictating to the body, what it 'thinks' or has been told it should do. It's about awareness of what is needed for body, mind and heart, trusting your own awareness to know what's best for you. Being taught or given guidance in these specific practices in the first place is useful, if not essential. It then needs to be made your own practice that evolves and changes over time according to your individual need and desire.

Neti

Before sitting for breathing practice, especially first thing in the morning, it is helpful to do a *kriya* (cleansing) yoga practice called *neti*. It is also called nasal irrigation.

You will need a pot with a spout and a good crystalline salt. There are several dedicated neti pots available online,* but a small indoor watering can with a narrow spout will be ok. Put a small amount of warm water into the pot and add some crystalline salt. How much salt you use is very individual, so begin with just a little. Too much could sting slightly; however, that does help the cleansing.

Stand over a sink, or do this outdoors if you prefer, as shown in the photo opposite. Hold the neti pot as shown there, and pour into one nostril or the other. The water may come out of that nostril or go across and come out of the other one: both will cleanse. After a few times of pouring change to the second

*For instance, there is one by the Himalayan Institute, available from www.iherb.com

KEN BELL

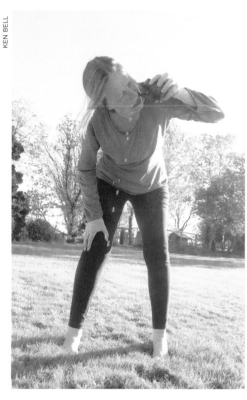

nostril. You can repeat each side two or three times until you feel the nostrils clearing.

It might take a few days or weeks completely to cleanse the nostrils. One you feel the cleansing is complete, you are best to continue two or three times a week – or to take a break of a week, as it can dehydrate the nose if you are using the salt generously.

Your *neti* routine will cleanse the nostrils and sinuses and down through the nasal passage, ready for all the following *pranayama*. It is helpful first to practice *kapabalati pranayama* as this will dry the nostrils. It is also very clearing during a cold or in similar conditions, especially at the first symptoms. Sometimes I have found that it can prevent infection like a cold developing. It can also be helpful for blocked sinuses and headaches, but needs perseverance.

Beginning *Pranayama* Practice

Follow the instructions for sitting in *parvatasana*, mountain pose (in chapter 3, which is the posture section for all of these pranayamas – see p. 77).

Rest your eyes and brain downwards to focus on the movement of the breath through the body. Feel how the floating ribs open above the strong, engaged first lumbar vertebra (see diagrams on pp 36, 40). This allows the breath to spread down to the lower part of the lungs, at the level of the floating ribs – and more towards the back of the body and out to the sides of the lung, forward and up to the top of the lungs.

Day by day, we tend not to access the lower part of the lungs as much as the upper. The lower lobes of the lungs connect more to the parasympathetic nervous system – which is the system that relaxes and calms us. The sympathetic nervous system, by contrast, is more connected to the upper lungs and is that part of the nervous system, which gets us up and doing. The sympathetic and parasympathetic nervous system are both part of the autonomic nervous system, which is what regulates and controls the internal organs unconsciously. The sympathetic nervous system – connected from the brain, via the cranial nerves, to the spine – controls the 'fight or flight' response to potentially dangerous situations. However, because we tend to use the upper lungs more than we use the lower lungs, the sympathetic nervous system becomes overstimulated, putting us under more or less constant stress, which in turn increases our heart rate and the tendency to rush about and not really able to relax easily.

The parasympathetic nervous system, by contrast, is connected to the cranial nerves via the vagus nerve and decreases the heart rate, increasing digestive hormones and so relaxes and calms the whole system. We obviously need a balance here, which can come about by using the the whole lungs. If you look at the diagram of the lungs repeated below from chapter 2, you will see that the trachea (windpipe) divides into the main left and right bronchus some way down the lungs. This is in order for the breath to spread down to the sides and up evenly. So by being consciously aware of this movement, which is increased by spreading the thoracic diaphragm and the lengthening of the lumbar spine, we can find that balance.

Overleaf (p. 87) I have set out a natural *pranayama*, a simple practice of breath awareness. Note that if you have not practised much *pranayama* before, it would be best to practise this natural *pranayama* regularly for some time, even a year or so, before going onto the others. There is a tendency to rush into powerful practices. However, this can put strain on the whole system, and the result is that we stop the practices and decide that they are not good for us. In fact, it is because we are trying to force too much too soon, when we have not engaged the spine in order to

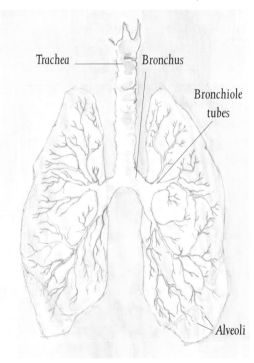

Trachea

Bronchus

Bronchiole tubes

Alveoli

change our posture. Deep healing usually takes time.

Pranayama also means awareness of the breath moving through the body, which gives a naturalness to breathing. Breathing *needs* to be completely natural. Often the term 'pranayama techniques' is used, but such a term implies forcing a technique onto a natural process.

These so-called techniques are actually natural ways of breathing *in certain circumstances*, when they are needed. So if we could be aware of how we breathe in the specific circumstances given below for each *pranayama*, it is very supportive to those circumstances – that is, the circumstances I've identified with each *pranayama.*

Pranayama techniques, when practised forcefully, can in fact be dangerous, and often people, especially cancer patients, are advized not to practise them. This is because there is a tendency to impose a forceful technique on top of a breathing pattern that is already under strain. The simple practice on the page opposite, beginning in *parvatasana*, mountain pose sitting, is about awareness of your breath only. It is not a technique but about becoming conscious of how you are already breathing. The body is a wonderful being, as it then finds over time a more natural breathing pattern, one that with awareness we can retain.

So it may be that you would need to only practise the simple *pranayama*, without force or strain (and for a very short time to begin with), or it may in itself be enough for you. It is enormous in and of itself. It does also need some awareness of posture first but it will gradually teach you this itself. As you become more aware of your breathing you will become more aware of your posture.

A Focus on the Breath

Begin your focus with the exhalation. As you exhale, keep the length of the spine forward and up towards the sky and spread across the shoulders, so that the exhalation sprays gently out. Wait at the end of the exhalation for your breath to come in again. Go with that movement in, to the top of the inhalation, and let it tumble over like a wave into the exhalation. Feel that although the mind can come in and take you off at a tangent, there is a rhythm to this that carries the mind along on the wave of the breath, like a wave of the sea, so that the mind can continually return to the movement of the breath through the body. Do this for as long as you can keep the focus, then see if you want to go on to a more specific *pranayama* as set out next.

You can feel that the breath lengthens and deepens purely from your total attention on it. You do not have to force or make it do this. The whole of the lungs will gradually fill from the bottom to the top and to the sides. This can then become a habit, day after day: to breathe more fully and slowly using the whole of the lungs. Yet this is not taking a forceful deep breath, as is often instructed, or pushing the air out. Remember to breathe always in and out through the the nose – that is what it is for – keeping your lips gently closed.

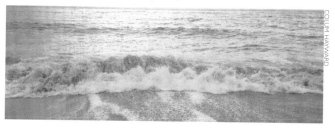

COLUM HAYWARD

Cleansing *Pranayama*

Kapabalati breath can be practised intentionally as a *pranay-ama*. This exhalation with short snorts is what we naturally do after running or in any way exerting the whole body. It cleanses the nostrils, sinuses and whole skull. *Kapabalati* is translated as 'shining skull' and it can have a wonderful effect.

Begin with *neti*. Nasal cleansing is particularly recommended for this *pranayama*.

Sitting with the spine lengthened forward and up and the shoulder girdle broadened and relaxed out, bring your awareness down to your breath, as it moves in and out through the nose. When you have settled into the rhythm of your breathing, breathe in through the nose, then breathe out through the nose in little snorts. Let the breath come in again, each time making a gentle snorting sound. Repeat this a few times.

Kapabalati breath is also helpful when we feel 'stuck' in mind or body in any way. Do not strain or overdo this breath – never 'go at it'. Stay with it only as long as your whole awareness is focused on your breathing, and then stop. A few breath-focused exhalations and inhalations are much more effective than forcing it.

How does it feel as you return to gentle inhalation and exhalation? Is there a sensation of clearing and a shining?

Nadi Sodhana

Nadi sodhana is generally translated as alternate nostril breathing, but this is a mistranslation. *Nadi* refers to the energy channels and *sodhana* means cleansing. So it's a cleansing of the 72,000 nadi or energy lines that travel through the body, rather like the meridians in acupuncture. However, the amount of flow through each nostril (not the direction of flow) does change throughout the day. You can be aware of this by bringing your attention to both nostrils. In the morning, generally the more active part of the day, the right nostril and right lung tend to bring more air in. In the evening, generally the more relaxing part of the day, the left nostril and lung tend to to bring more air in. However, this can continually change through the day, depending on what the mind and body are doing.

You might like to contemplate the connection of brain to nostril in your investigation and practice. The left side of the body is linked to the right side of the brain and the right side of the body is linked to the left side of the brain. So the left nostril is linked to the right side of the brain and the right nostril is linked to the left side of the brain.

Iain McGilchrist, who wrote the book THE MASTER AND HIS EMISSARY on the subject, is the great authority on the two sides of the brain, a subject that was somewhat misunderstood when it first becoame popular. It is a very big book to read, but in the TED talk, 'The Divided Brain and the Search for Meaning', McGilchrist gives some clarity on these two sides of the brain, firstly in animals and birds, who have this same division.*

When a bird is looking for seeds on the ground it needs a focused attention to pick out the seeds from the earth. This is more the domain of the left hemisphere of the brain. But the bird also needs to be vigilant with a broad vision looking out for predators. This is the domain of the right hemisphere, also needed when looking out for a mate (there is a correlation with the peripheral and predator types of vision described by Bridget on pp 64-7).

*See 'Further Reading' for full references to both book and talk

In humans, similarly, the left hemisphere of the brain gives a more sharply focused attention, while the right hemisphere a sustained, alert, broad, open and vigilant connection to the world.

Albert Einstein is recorded as saying.

'The intuitive mind is a sacred gift,

'The reasoning mind is a faithful servant.

'We have created a soul that honours the servant but has forgotten the gift.'

It feels to me that the right hemisphere is more about how we really feel and think and the left hemisphere is more about how we think we should feel and think. I have come over many years to practise this *pranayama* by simply being aware of how the breath comes into each nostril and into the two sides of the lungs. My reason for talking about the two sides of the brain is that we can use our breath awareness to nourish and balance the brain, too.

So, lying down or sitting, become aware which side feels fuller and then focus there for a few breaths. And then come to the side that feels not so full, the ribs and nostril not opening as much, and see if the attention there encourages more opening there.

This is very subtle and takes patience and perseverance rather than the forceful way *nadi sodhana* is sometimes taught – which is by closing one nostril with the fingers and so forcing all the breath through one nostril. The nostrils are very fine, delicate instruments of the body and do not respond well to this forceful treatment. Fine capillary blood vessels in the lining of the nose can be damaged and the cilia (the fine cleansing hairs) can be affected, so that they are not able to do their cleansing job so well.

If you lie on your left side, do you feel that the right nostril opens more? It is a custom in India to lie on the left side after a meal as stimulating the right lung helps the stimulation of the digestive fires. The Sanskrit word *agni* refers to these 'digestive fires' and is important in ayurvedic medicine. The right side is more connected to the warming and stimulating sympathetic nervous system.

What happens if you then lie on your right side? Is the left nostril open more? This is better for inducing sleep, as it is more connected to the calming and cooling parasympathetic nervous system.

Remember that from the beginning of this chapter we have also been working with how the sympathetic nervous system is more linked to the top of the lungs (where we tend to breathe most) and the bottom area of the lungs (not used so much) is more linked to the parasympathetic nervous system.

After *nadi sohana*, you could then continue to:

Chandra bedhana pranayama

In the name *chandra bedhana pranayama*, 'chandra' is the moon and relates to the left nostril's calming energy. '*Bedhana*' means passing through.

After noticing the difference in the nostrils from *nadi sodhana* you can feel which nostril needs to open more – or what you yourself at that time wish to stimulate. If it's a calming quietening energy for relaxation and sleep, lying or sitting, then consciously breathing in through the left and out through the left lung and nostril may be useful. Notice the effect of that as you come back to breathing through both nostrils.

I never teach students to close the nostrils forcefully. The best

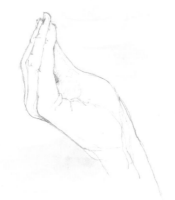

way is with the lotus mudra shown in the photo. Close all the fingers to the thumb (first drawing, which shows the right hand). As you inhale, gradually open the fingers (second photo) like a lotus or a tulip opening up. Can you feel that that would bring the breath in more through the left nostril? As you exhale, let the left fingers close, feeling that the breath goes out through the left nostril more.

If the left nostril feels very blocked, put a finger on your *right* c h e e k b o n e

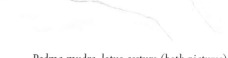

Padma mudra, lotus gesture (both pictures)

and ease a little to the right. Can you feel that the breath going through the left nostril then goes across and relaxes the right hemisphere of the brain more? This will be expanded on in chapter 8.

Regular practice will bring much more sensitivity to the nostrils and their connection to the brain, so that in time you will be able to feel immediately which nostril is dominant at any one time, or which feels more appropriate. For the right nostril:

Surya bedhana pranayama

Here you do the opposite: breathe in through the right nostril first and then out through the right to stimulate a more active energy. Again, breathe easily in and out after a few breaths to notice the effect of this practice. Can you sense that

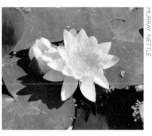

the breath coming through the right nostril then goes across and relaxes the left hemisphere of the brain more?

In time and with a regular practice you should be able to notice this difference at any time of day, and then focus more on one nostril than the other as you breathe, if you wish to balance them or stimulate one or the other.

Relaxing and Calming Pranayama

How often, when concentrating on doing something delicate, enjoyable, important do we tend to hum? Does it help the concentration?

Bhramari (Humming Bee) breath with Khechari mudra

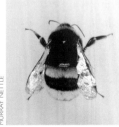

This supports and enhances our concentration. Maybe that is why a bee makes such a hum with its wings it when collecting nectar? This breath can be practised with *khechari mudra*, the word 'mudra' sometimes being translated as a gesture.

Khechari mudra is when the tongue rolls up and back so the tip and some of the back of the tongue are firm on the roof of the mouth. This makes the mouth fuller, so the humming sound is more of a traditional hum and louder. *Khechari mudra* translates as 'space walking seal'; it also means 'attitude of dwelling in supreme consciousness'.

Instructions

1.   Sit with the spine lengthening forward and up from the base of the spine to the crown of the head, so the head is balanced on top of the atlas bone and the shoulder girdle is broadening out to the side.

2.   Focus your awareness on gently breathing in and out through your nose for a few minutes.

3.   Roll the tip of your tongue up and back towards the roof of your mouth. Keep it there in *khechari mudra*.

4.   Keeping your lips shut and your teeth a little apart, breathe in fully through your nose. As you breathe out make a humming sound like a female bee. Feel that the sound fills your whole mouth, strong and sonorous. Continue for several breaths, noticing if the sound gets stronger.

5.   Rest, breathe easily, and feel the effects of it. Notice if, with regular practice, it has any of the effects given below.

According to the *Hatha Yoga Pradipika*, the ancient text, this breath relieves stress, anger, anxiety and insomnia. It strengthens the voice and clears and alleviates throat ailments. It's helpful to practise in labour. The *Pradipika*, setting out these benefits, is the earliest writing on *hatha yoga*.

Viloma, the Ladder Breath

Letting-go Breath: on the exhalation

1.   Sit with the spine forward and up and bring your attention to your breathing so that it naturally lengthens and

deepens for a few minutes.

2.   Then on the next exhalation breathe out a little and pause, then breathe out again and pause. Continue until you feel you have breathed right out (which we very often do not do).

3.   Let the breath come in again when it is ready – easily and gently.

4.   Then repeat the pauses on the exhalation for three to five breaths. On a daily practice of *pranayama*, you can slowly increase the number of pauses.

Does this relax you? Would you do it naturally if you become aware that you are not breathing right out?

Stimulating Breath: on the inhalation

Important: you should have regularly practised viloma on the exhalation before going onto the inhalation, so that you are relaxed.

1.   Sit with the spine lengthened, bringing your full attention to your breath for a few minutes.

2.   After an exhalation, breathe in a little and pause. Then inhale again and pause as the lungs gradually fill from the bottom upwards, until you reach the top of the inhalation. Then exhale completely.

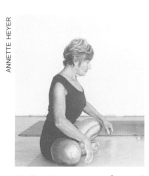

ANNETTE HEYER

Sophy Hoare sitting forward and up for Viloma

3.   Repeat for three to five breaths to start with, allowing the number to increase naturally over time. However, it is important not to overdo the numbers of breaths you take like this. It is not a set routine of physical practice but a mindful awareness of breathing. So if we overdo it, the mind goes off somewhere else and we stop practising, and then we push and strain.

A pause is not a holding of the breath. One of my yoga teachers, Sophy Hoare, would say 'breathe in, and breathe in, then breathe in again', emphasizing the ladder-like awareness so that there is no tightening or strain.

Does pausing on the inhalation feel energizing? Would you do this naturally if you felt that you had not breathed in enough?

Stimulating and Focusing *Pranayama*

Ujjayi pranayama

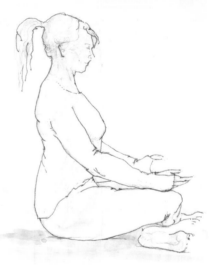

'Ujjayi' means victorious, so this *pranayama* conquers unwanted mind states. When we need to gather ourselves together for something important – to say something significant, to be at our best at a special occasion, a speech, an interview, and so on – what do we do with our body? There is the expression, 'She gathered herself up to her full height'. Does this remind you of *tadasana* (p. 58)? By raising ourselves up, by practising *tadasana*, does our breath naturally deepen, lengthen? Are we more conscious of it coming in and going out? I find myself standing like this before a long drive or a meeting.

If we could follow this effect in the breath more specifically in *ujjayi pranayama* it would give us good support on those occasions, since it is at once steadying and enlivening.

1.   When you are preparing for the special occasion, need energizing, or you feel for any reason at all the need to practise this *pranayama*, give yourself five or ten minutes to sit with the spine lengthened forward and up and be aware of how you are breathing first. Does your breath naturally deepen? If so, go with that movement so that it increases, but not forcefully.

2.   Then, at the top of the inhalation, feel the lift up under the top of the breastbone; enhance that a little by pausing there (just pausing, not holding) and lifting a little more. Does the head surrender down to the heart? Let this happen naturally rather than dropping the head. It can be an almost imperceptible movement of the head and a resting and broadening back of the whole throat area. See the picture on the previous page.

3.   Exhale whenever you feel ready to. Let the breath come in again. Let the ribs open to the side and back so the whole of the lungs fill. The head will return gently to its upright position as the breath comes in. This usually just needs a few breaths to bring about a sense of being 'ready for anything'.

Ujjayi with Khumbaka Breath:

Retention on the Inhalation
If you would like or need this *ujjayi pranayama* to be more stimulating, follow the instructions given above, but at the top of the inhalation pause with the breath in and then go on lifting and opening the top of the chest to the side, at the back and at the front.

Only pause for as long as you are lifting and opening. This

will probably be a very short time at first but will extend with practice. Exhale gently and slowly when your body feels ready.

If the breath rushes out after the retention, it means that you have held it too long and too forcefully. So find a balance, as always, between the inhalation and exhalation by not breathing in too forcefully or holding on too long.

Repeat this a few times without overdoing it. A few quality focused breaths are better than allowing it to become too much of a routine. Sit for a few minutes or longer to feel the effect of *ujjayi pranayama* on mind, body, breath and spirit.

Khumbaka is translated as breath retention. If this is practised by a forceful holding of the breath in, it can cause disturbance and strain. It is better therefore to consider the so-called 'hold' as a pause, just as before. There is less likelihood then of a tightening and contracting in the body and mind. I have always been wary of holding the breath, as many of the instructions you come across are about forcefully tightening, to stop either at the end of the exhalation or the inhalation, which puts a strain everywhere in the body and mind.

People hold their breath in their sleep when they suffer from sleep apnoea. There is now what is termed 'email apnoea' – when we have so many channels of social media that we can go to and fro from one to another to the extent that we forget to breathe – and we also forget what we have just done! This is incredibly common now, but it is still unconsciously holding your breath, which is obviously detrimental to your whole body and mind.

Consciously pausing at certain specific points in a specific *pranayama* breathing rhythm is a very different thing, and needs years of a regular breathing practice before we are ready to approach it, together with an upright spine and lungs that can fully fill. Only forty-two years on from having been taught the above stimulating *ujjayi* breath with the pausing and continued lifting by Sri B.K.S. Iyengar in India do I now feel ready to explore *khumbaka* in a more relaxed way, with a slow build-up.

Retention on the Exhalation

1.   Follow the deepening of the breath given in the second paragraph of this chapter for about at least five minutes.

2.   Then, at the end of the next exhalation pause with the breath right out for as long as feels comfortable to do so – being aware that this will increase with each breath, and with each new practice of this pause at the end of the exhalation.

3.   Feel how the breath comes in now, deeply and strongly. Exhale and repeat for as long as your focus can stay with it, noticing any difference with each exhalation.

4.   Then return to gently breathing in and breathing out, noticing how you feel.

There is currently much research around retention of the breath. Scientists have, for instance, investigated the ability of the Dutchman Wim Hof to withstand cold after breathing exercises.* The research conducted on him found that the body chemistry changed from acid to alkaline in the course of his breath retention, because more carbon dioxide is eliminated in that pause. Carbon dioxide is acidic in nature and we can tend to retain too much if we don't breathe right out.

Such a change in the body chemistry from acid to alkaline would also happen in the Viloma breath, particularly on the exhalation – which needs to be practised many times before any retention of the breath). There are potential health benefits from this change in the body chemistry too.†

*See his book , THE WIM HOF METHOD
†go to www.healthline.com//respiratoryalkalosisandacidosis for detailed information on respiratory acidosis and alkalosis

Bhastrika Breath

This is a very stimulating breath that needs full and regular practice of both *kapabalati* and *ujjayi* breath for some time, even years, beforehand. It has taken me twenty years of regular practice of those breaths before I feel that I can approach *bastrika* without force.

Bastrika means bellows, which are used to stimulate a fire to get it to burn more strongly. For this reason, *bastrika* is sometimes called the Breath of Fire – as it stimulates your own 'inner fire-energy'. This is the stimulation of the *kundalini* energy, which resides between the base of the spine and the sacrum and is likened to a coiled serpent. Much is said about the stimulation of this *kundalini* energy – its effects and its dangers. In my experience it feels very linked to *prana* – the natural life force within us. The physical body in yoga is known as the *ana-maya-kosa*. *Maya* means illusion (that which changes is 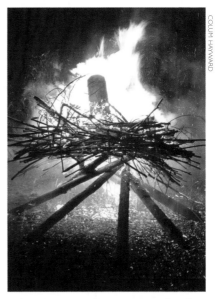 illusionary). *Kosa* is a layer or covering and *ana* means food so it is the body that needs sustaining with food.

The more subtle level of the body is the *prana-maya-kosa* – the body that needs sustaining with the life force that comes from the air we breathe. The link between these two bodies is considered to be between the base of the spine and the sacrum, where the kundalini power resides.

The movement at this level of the pelvic floor diaphragm, in junction with the thoracic diaphragm to bring the breath in, is a very vital part of breathing, and stimulates the energy all the way up the spine and into the lungs and circulatory system. It thus gives increased vitality, energy, resilience. This is the *kundalini* energy.

Instructions for Bhastrika

1.   Sit with the spine lengthened forward and up with your focus on the breath coming in going out.

2.   When you feel settled and have focused on your breathing for around five minutes, practise a few rounds of *kapabalati* – little snorts on the exhalation (full instructions were given under cleansing breaths, p. 88).

3.   Then breathe in fast, breathe out fast, eight or ten times.

4.   Take a few regular breaths.

5.   Then repeat the fast breath in and the fast breath out ten or twelve times. A bit faster or a bit longer than the previous sequence if possible. This is enough for the first few times of practice.

6.   Really notice the effects of this practice. The speed of breathing will increase as you go on.

Bellows are used to stimulate fire. That's the effect of this practice over time: to generate your own inner fire in the belly, and it to be able to move it up through the the spine so it can produce a lot of heat and be very cleansing, and then settle down in the heart area, to enable yourself to focus on love and warmth.

When does this bellows breath happen naturally in life? During orgasm? During childbirth? Both are times of very heightened awareness. I was aware of it both at the conceiving and during the birth of my daughter – having conceived my only child when I was forty, having been told that I could not conceive.

Yoga teacher Angela Farmer says of this breath that 'it unlocks holding patterns' so it could be accompanied by some shaking vibration throughout the whole body and warmth in different places.

I have experienced warm tingling in my hands for about two weeks after doing *bhastrika*, which others could feel when they touched my hands, and a significant shift of mind and emotional states,which can relieve depression and anxiety.

There is an adaption of *bhastrika*, adopted from India by Tibetan Buddhists, called Tummo breathing, which has been kept more secret for thousands of years. However it is now a popular practice in some parts of the world. It is more forceful, as the exhalation is strongly pushed out through the mouth, accompanied by a strong movement forward of the whole trunk, and therefore the effects can be stronger and accompanied by profuse sweating, headaches and feeling very faint.

It is for those who want a very strong shift in themselves and their lives, and it needs to be taught by an experienced and compassionate teacher. I am very unsure of the wisdom of pushing the breath forcefully through the mouth.

The regular practice of these sitting pranayamas will gradually bring more awareness of how we breathe generally day to day. And so it will become more natural – and we will thus find the rhythm and balance we need.

Chapter 5 : Breathing and the Feelings

*'The process of breathing, if we can begin to understand it
in relation to the whole of life , shows us the way to let go of
the old and open to the new.'*
Dennis Lewis, THE TAO OF NATURAL BREATHING

THIS CHAPTER is about how feelings, emotions and mind
states affect the breathing and how awareness of breathing can
relieve strained mind states, anxiety and depression.

When you feel states of mind that can be overwhelming
and troubling it is initially very helpful to pause and notice
how those states affect how you are breathing. If you can do
something about your breathing, then you can relieve an unhelpful mind state. Really all that's needed is to be constantly
aware of how you are breathing.

Anxiety

In anxiety, there is a tendency to hold the breath in. Consciously breathe out through your nose. Wait. Let your breath
come gently and fully in, without force, and then consciously
breathe out in stages (this is *viloma*, the ladder breath, given
in the *pranayama* section)

Exhale a little, pause; exhale again, pause – until you feel
that you have breathed right out without pushing. Wait for
the breath to find its own way in. Do this until the anxiety
subsides. However, do not overdo so that it becomes mechanical: your whole attention needs to be with your breathing.

Depression

In depression there is a tendency to hold the breath out, literally depressing the whole system. Can you become aware
of this tendency first, and of how it collapses your posture ?

Consciously take a breath in, gently breathe out, then wait.
Feel that the breath wants to come in. Can you let it do so
gently and easily, and can you let it fill the lungs of its own
accord? Go with this movement until the breath comes and
goes easily and your spirits lift. It is good to go for a walk while
you are doing this.

You may feel that this would not work for severe or clini-
cal depression. Certainly, it would be more difficult and there
would likely be a reluctance to try.

This is a long-term healing process to be used alongside
other therapies and would need to be practised regularly at the
times when the depression is not so severe.

Strain and Stress

When you are feeling under strain or otherwise stressed there
is again a tendency to hold the breath. Conscious breathing
and either of the practices just described will take you out of
that strain. It is not always easy or comfortable to focus on
breathing as it is so intimately connected with how we feel so
it can be good to start with posture.

The standing posture used to start a yoga practice, *tadasana*, is usually called 'Mountain pose' – however, as I explained
earlier, the Sanskrit actually means 'As it is now'. 'As it is now'
changes from moment to moment and within a yoga practice
from one posture to the next. See if you can be aware of this in
your day-to-day life, in standing, walking and in your practice.

So, when you can, focus on standing – in bare feet and outside if possible. Spread down into the Earth through your feet (notice the roots shown in the picture). Does this have the effect of bringing your breath in? Now, can the thighbones stand up more in to the hip socket? – so that the spine goes forward and up, through the shoulders, which then broaden and relax the whole shoulder girdle out. The crown of the head can then come in line with the coccyx, the base of the spine.

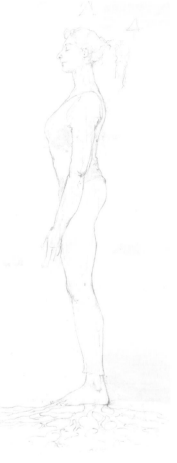

What happens when you breathe out? Do the feet make more contact with the ground and yet the spine goes on lengthening and waking up? Can you stay here for several breaths to give you a connection to the Earth energy and so a trust in the earth to support you with whatever is going on in your life? Also, can the Earth give you a sense of security?

From your firm contact through your feet is there a sense of a security in that contact that is not there in the world that we live in – much as we try to make it so through money, relationships, homes, insurances? This lack of security has been very evident during the pandemic, hasn't it?

Standing with this focus would be a great help for anxiety, stress, depression, lack of confidence.

The Skandhas

The Buddha described as pairs of opposites the worldly concerns that are common to us all and lead to the conditions just described:

Praise/Blame: how much do we look for praise and endorsement of ourselves? What happens when we get blame or criticism? We are so affected by both, aren't we? Could we practise learning from them without going into a big reaction to either?

Gain/Loss. These crop up throughout our lives. How can we go with this fluctuation, knowing that the situation will constantly change?

Success/Failure. This starts when we are young, especially when being taught at school, and becomes very prevalent in the business and sport world. Can we go with accepting both evenly?

Fame/Disrepute. I am very aware as a 'yoga teacher' that I can be put on a pedestal and am aware of doing that to others – but we always fall off that pedestal at some time.

The Buddha talked about how we cling to these worldly concerns, each of which gives us a craving for what we see as the good aspects, and gave the principles of the Skandhas to support us in becoming aware of this transitory nature of our existence here. These principles form one of the most important teachings of the Buddha. The Sanskrit word is *skandhas*, and the Pali (the Buddhist form of writing) is *khandhas*. Both mean heaps, collections, aggregates or groupings. It refers to the five material and mental factors that are part of the arising of craving and clinging, which we'll now explore. The Buddha considered that this clinging and craving causes our suffering.

There is a great deal to contemplate here, when we are challenged by a difficult or debilitating mind state. Perhaps we can consider what we may be expecting out of life and our journey on this planet in order to begin understanding why the Lord Buddha states this?

The Five Skandhas which we tend to create as a response to our fears are:

1.   *Bodily formations.* Formations are *samskaras* in Sanskrit, *sankaras* in Pali. This is where the body tightens in response to a situation, feeling or a mental proliferation*. We can feel this as we sit, stand, walk and focus on the body and

---

* *In the Buddha's teaching, 'mental proliferation' describes how we allow the mind to go on and on from one thing to another, and more precisely the process by which we are led on to the next thought. For example, the idea of catching Covid-19 leads us to anxiety, and in turn we imagine being in hospital, not being able to catch our breath, coughing constantly, dying. It is not helpful to allow the mind to go on a hypothetical track like that, however real it may feel to our imagination. It is possible to breathe through a proliferation, consciously going with the exhalation, so that it extends and goes right out – without pushing it – and then letting the breath come in. But don't extend or force it in any way.*

Notice whether you can trace back to where the disturbing thought began, and so let it go. I find this most helpful as it does seem to go naturally if you find the origin of the thought while in the awareness of breathing. This Buddhist practice is not easy. You will need to do it over and over for the rest of your life here on Earth! – but it can be done with attention and discipline, and it will allow us to take charge of our own lives.

the breath going in and going out. (See chapter 7, on Mind-fulness and Meditation). The most common places to tighten are the jaw, the teeth, the tongue, the throat, the brow, the shoulders and the fists, often accompanied by holding our breath. If we can relax these bodily formations that will have a great effect on the mind state and how we are breathing.

Remember that essentially the state of the mind is not who we are as it is constantly changing. If we can let go, then we can become aware of the natural mind state, *citta* in Sanskrit (see p. 123), which can allow us to come to the place where we realise just how much 'we change our mind'.

2.   *Feeling formations.* How we feel and respond to a sit-uation or to other people changes moment by moment. If we can be aware of this in any moment and any situation we can perhaps let it not take us over. The Buddhist concept of the impermanence of everything is really helpful here.

I know there can be very drastic and terrible situations that we can find ourselves in, and these can cause powerful post-traumatic stress. Such conditions are much more difficult to handle in this way, but over time and with support and instruction this approach would be very healing. The same principle of relaxing and letting go as in the first skandha is helpful – with a particular focus on breathing slowly so that the exhalation lengthens and lets go.

3.   *Perception formations.* This is our view of ourselves, others, and the world with all its opinions, which again are subject to tremendous change often according to the infor-mation we receive, assume and understand, which will change our perception minute by minute. Again, if we can be aware of this and our body's response to it and how it affects how we breathe, the perceptions we have can begin to let go their hold on us.

4.   *Mind formations.* These are also known as mind objects, mind transitions, mental proliferations. This is where the mind goes off on a journey into the past or into speculation, planning and preoccupation with the future. This is the most powerful *skandha* and the hardest to stop. In fact, we are not trying to stop it, but to become aware of it, and we need to be aware that that is happening and breathe throughout it. A slow exhalation two to four seconds longer than the inhalation is helpful.

5.   *Sense consciousness.* Awareness of the senses can cause all of the first four. Imagine if we are meditating, relaxing, sitting, breathing, walking, practising our yoga, and a good smell of food comes along. What particular smell would that be for you? Vegetables cooking? Coffee on the go? Chocolate? A delicious cheese? The senses will take us off in all directions: memories of having enjoyed a particularly good piece of cheese in France, a great cup of coffee in Italy, a lovely meal with friends at home. They are good memories but they distract us from what we are doing and lead us off into all the other formations – unless we realise how hungry or thirsty we are and go to have whatever we crave! If, of course, we are 'lucky' enough to be in a position to do that.

Chapter 6 : Chanting

Why Chant?

SANSKRIT IS thought to be the oldest original language our current global civilization has developed. It has a particular resonant sound and is considered to have evolved from a time when people in the Indus Valley of India looked at nature and felt a vibration from it – and then made a sound that resonated with that vibration. This may seem difficult for material minds to understand or accept, but because those people lived much closer to nature than we do now they were much more sensitive. Rather like the ancient civilization that built Stonehenge five or six thousand years ago (thought now to be around the same time as the Indus Valley civilization) people of these early cultures also had a highly sensitive awareness of the sky and the rhythm of the Sun and the Moon – to the extent that Stonehenge is now seen as a highly evolved map of these movements with an astonishing accuracy. As this book is written there are new discoveries about Stonehenge that show an entire circle of stones was moved from the Preseli Hills in West Wales, already dressed and standing, to the Stonehenge site. We can only speculate why, but it is worth noting our tendency to think that we are more evolved than our ancestors. It may be a dangerous arrogance!

There is also speculation that they would have chanted as they moved these extremely heavy stones. Did that chanting lighten the load? Paramahansa Yogananda apparently stated that the vibration of the chant synchronized with the vibration of the stones and did literally lighten them, and the spiritual

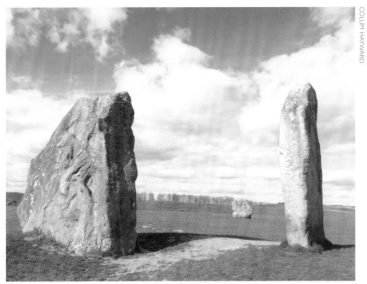

COLUM HAYWARD

Standing stones at Avebury, Wiltshire

teacher White Eagle also talks of sound as being involved in their movement. And in the same way the walls of Jericho fell.

Was this 'entrainment'? Entrainment, in the bio-musico-logical sense, refers to the synchronization of organisms to an external perceived rhythm such as human music and dance. Humans are said to be the only species within which all individuals experience entrainment, although there are documented examples in non-human species such as in the sea lion.

Everything has a vibration, all living beings certainly, but also rocks, crystals, the sea, sand, clouds and so on. You only need to look at the latest nature programmes on television to see how all of these are gradually being accepted as living beings now.

Vedic chanting is the most ancient form of chanting that we at present know about. It has traditionally been part of the practice of yoga, as it harmonizes the energy channels, called nadis. Ancient Vedic chanting was handed down through generations by listening to the subtle sounds heard, and then repeating them with the same tone and resonance. This resonance has a deep effect on the whole system and on how you breathe. It regulates the breath and the heart rate and that harmonizes the whole system.

When you start to learn Vedic chanting in Sanskrit it very specifically focuses on 'yoga for the mouth', which is designed to exercise the muscles and to be able to open the mouth wide. This consists not only of widening the mouth but also moving the jaws from side to side and making all sorts of funny faces! Then the focus is on the pronunciation of each and every letter and sound. Only after some considerable practice of these is the chanting, such as the sutras of Patanjali, taught.

Resonance Breathing

It is a yoga principle that the slowing of your breathing rate increases health and longevity. Singing, and particularly chanting, do the same thing. *Pranayama* – awareness of breathing – is another way to achieve it.

The average breathing rate for an adult is fifteen to eighteen breaths a minute. When I am breathing mindfully, I count as few as eight breaths per minute. With a pause at the end of an exhalation, the rate that I counted is between five and six breaths a minute – that is, between ten and twelve seconds per full breath.

There seems to be something significant about this rate of

To read in more detail and have instruction go to www.the-wholenessofyoga.com/vedic-chanting. Sarah Waterfield, who will be contacted via that site, was my own teacher and works with the Inner Yoga School.

breathing and a number of studies correlate its significance. For instance, when the yoga sutra of Patanjali, no. 1.2 – 'Yoga is the settling of the mind into silence' – is chanted in Sanskrit silently on the inhalation and out loud on the exhalation, it is reckoned to take 5.5 seconds for each inhalation and each exhalation. In Sanskrit, the chant is *Yogah citta vritti nirodhah.*

If the tongue is put into *khechari mudra* on the roof of the mouth then the inhalation has been observed to take 5.5 seconds and the exhalation also 5.5 seconds.

The yoga and Tibetan Buddhist mantra *Om Mani Padme Hum*, which translates as 'the jewel in the heart of the lotus', also takes 5.5 seconds.

Comparisons have been made with the sections of the *Ave Maria*, chanted in Latin, although the whole chant there is longer. The University of Pavia in Italy conducted experiments on the chanting of *Ave Maria* and found that average number of breaths for each cycle of chant by the priest and the response by the nuns was six seconds (see the link below*).

Https://www.ncbi.nlm.nih.gov/pmc/articles/PMC61046

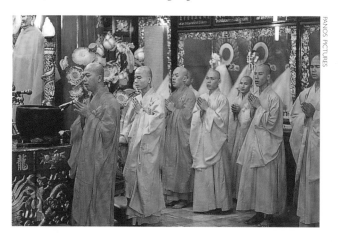

PANOS PICTURES

There is a connection here: the rosary, which may be used alongside the chanting of the Ave Maria, was introduced into Europe by the Arabs who in turn took it from the Tibetan monks, who took it from the yoga Masters of India.

An online article by Olga Kabel compares the rhythm of the heart and the blood pressure to this breathing rate.* Although work remains to be done, the outcome of these fascinating investigations seems to be that if our breathing rate is slowed to about six breaths per minute there is a resonance with heart rate variability (Mayer) and with the regulation of blood pressure – known as baroreflex sensitivity – and also with the nervous system. Here is James Nestor again, whom we cited earlier in the book as a recent writer on the breath:

> 'It turned out that the most efficient breathing rhythm occurred when both the length of respirations and total breaths

* *www.sequencewiz.org//what is your optimal breathing rate and why it matters*

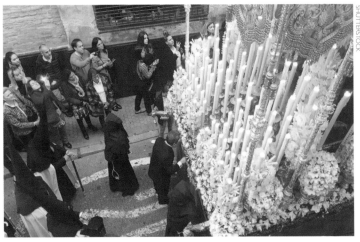

per minute were locked into a spooky symmetry: 5.5 second inhales followed by 5.5 second exhales, which works out almost exactly to 5.5 breaths a minute.'*

This is termed 'resonant' or 'coherent' breathing.

Is this resonance why it feels so good to chant in this specific way, with the strong focus on the pronunciation and the movement of the mouth, and why it feels inspiring and relaxing to listen to the *Ave Maria* in Latin?? Does it connect us more to the parasympathetic nervous system? Or to some source outside of ourselves – 'the unmanifest' – known as Brahma in the Vedas: *that which cannot be known*?

It is a much slower rate of breathing than the normal average rate. I have tried to show in this book that this is because in our busy lives and with our somewhat sunken posture we are using mostly the top part of the lungs, so we then need to breathe at a faster rate. So the sympathetic nervous system is overstimulated, and that is responsible for 'getting us going'. The trouble is, once we 'start up' in this way it is highly difficult to stop!

There are a thousand ways now to relax, and some of them quite expensive. Why can't we do it by focusing on our breathing, which is free?

'Everything around us is pulsating and vibrating-nothing is really standing still.

'The Om sound, when chanted vibrates at 432 Hertz, which is the same vibrational frequency as everything in nature. As such, AUM is the basic sound as everything in nature, so by chanting it we are symbolically and physically acknowledging our connection to nature and all other living beings.'

Sam Saunders (www.mindbodygreen.com)

BREATH, p. 83

The *Om* Sound

> *'The Om sound mystically embodies the*
> *essence of the whole universe.'*
>
> ENCYCLOPAEDIA BRITANNICA

When I was first taught chanting in Sanskrit I was instructed to put three fingers in line on top of one another so that the mouth opens very wide to make the O sound of the *OM* or *AUM*. This took quite a bit of doing but it did make for a clear sound. It must also help the shaping of the mouth in the way described by the orthodontist Mike Mew, which we saw on p. 49!

The AUM sound has three separate sounds in it:

• The 'A' – pronounced short like the 'e' in 'her', is sounded with the mouth as wide open as possible, hence the three fingers in the mouth!

• the 'U' sound – (pronounced as in 'put') has the same full wide mouth with the teeth coming closer together (but still space between them) to create UUUU.

• the 'M' sound is still full in the mouth, teeth apart still, but lips lightly closed (pronounced as 'Me' in 'merchant')

These are sounded separately several times, then put together by only changing the shape of the mouth – breathing in through the nose and out through both nose and mouth. The sound eventually becomes a continuous AUM or OOOM sound that can continue for quite a while and has the effect of clearing the mind. It is traditionally chanted at the beginning of meditation to settle the mind into *samadhi* (translated as the settled mind, the third stage of meditation) and sometimes at the end to signal the end of the meditation.

The Mandukya Upanishad

The significance of the Aum is thus described in the Upanishads, the later Vedic texts. The Mandukya or Mandooka Upanishad is dated somewhere in the two centuries before the Common (Christian) Era. We read:

'The self is the lord of all; inhabitant of the hearts of all.

'This Self, although beyond words, is that supreme word Om; though indivisible, it can be divided in three letters corresponding to the three conditions of the self, the letter A, the letter U and the letter M.

'The waking condition, called the material condition, corresponds to the letter A, which leads the alphabet and breathes in all the other letters. He who understands this, gets all he wants; becomes a leader amongst men.

'The dreaming condition, called the mental condition, corresponds to the second letter U. It upholds; stands between waking and sleeping. He who understands, upholds the tradition of spiritual knowledge; looks upon everything with an impartial eye.

'No one ignorant of spirit is born into this family.

'Undreaming sleep, called the intellectual condition, corresponds to the third letter M. It weighs and unites. Those who understand, weigh the world; reject; unite themselves with the cause.

'The fourth condition of the self corresponds to Om as one indivisible word. He/she is whole beyond bargain. The world disappears in them. They are the good. Thus Om is nothing but Self. Those who understand, with the help of the personal self, merge into the impersonal Self; those who understand.'

THE TEN PRINCIPAL UPANISHADS, translated
by Shree Purohit Swami and W. B. Yeats

The regulation and resonance the chanting gives are very helpful and important for the regulation and rhythm of breathing. If we get into the rhythm of the chanting with regular practice this will gradually give more rhythm to our breathing pattern, returning it to a more natural way. Also, the meaning of the chants can have some significance for us – which encourages the chant and so encourages the ease of breathing.

Here, now, are some regular chants.

The Perfect Prayer

'That is perfect. This is perfect. Perfect comes from perfect.
'Take perfect from perfect, the remainder is perfect.
'May peace and peace and peace be everywhere.'
> *Eesha (or Isa) Upanishad, put into English by Shree Purohit Swami and W. B. Yeats*

In Sanskrit this is:

> *Om purna madaha*
> *purna madacyate*
> *purnosya purnamevava sisyate*
> *Om santih santih santih.*

Also translated as 'wholeness', this chant is traditionally chanted when things in this earthly life do not feel perfect or whole in order for us to come to acceptance of how things are.

The three repetitions of peace (*santih, santih, santih* in Sanskrit) mean:

First time – peace within ourselves.

Second time – peace within our immediate environment and those we are in regular contact with.

Third – peace within the greater whole, the world, the universe.

The Teacher's Prayer

This chant is often used in yoga classes.

'May we be protected (the teacher and the student).
'May we enjoy teaching and learning.
'May we teach and learn wholeheartedly and thus gain insight and clarity.
'May there be no enmity between us.
'May there be peace within us, around us and far from us.'

*Taitreeya Upanishad, put into English
by Shree Purohit Swami and W. B. Yeats*

In Sanskrit:

*Om Saha navavatu
Saha Nadu bhunaktu
Saha biryanis karavavahai
Ma vidvisavahai
Om Santih santih santih.*

Chapter 7 : Mindfulness

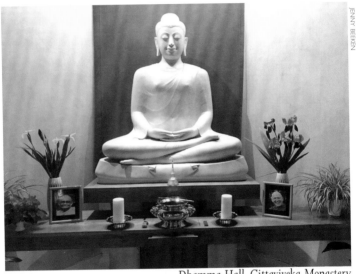

Dhamma Hall, Cittaviveka Monastery

'Breathing in, I know that I am breathing in.
'Breathing out, I know that I am breathing out.'

Thich Nhat Hanh

IN ORDER to breathe easily and naturally through the nose and then begin to use the whole of the lungs and main respiratory muscles, we only need to become aware of breathing in and breathing out. If we do this without trying or interfering with the breath in any way, it will return to the natural rhythm that it can all too easily lose in our daily life. This is mindfulness of breathing, taught originally by the Buddha.

We can do this any time of the day or night whilst standing, sitting, walking, running, resting, gardening, swimming, working out, thinking. It's extremely helpful while thinking! It would also help the transition to sleep.

This is the mindfulness of living: being a human being rather that a human doing.

All of the practices I've discussed will settle the mind, albeit briefly in some cases. But brevity is alright, as it brings an awareness of the effect we can have on the day-to-day mind while allowing it to go where it will – yet with the awareness that there is another aspect of mind. That is the natural mind, which is in tune with the natural world and natural breathing (see the Buddha's 'Mindfulness of Breathing' below); in tune with the natural rhythms.

This recognition will prevent us from beating ourselves up about 'not being able to do mindfulness or meditation'. It is not the point, to judge ourselves in this way, but will help us commit ourselves to purely sitting with ourselves as we are without any judgment of how we are doing – an enormous change from how we usually judge ourselves and what we do.

Vedic philosophy offers four aspects of mind: *buddhi, citta, manas* and *ahamkara. Ahamkara*, in Sanskrit, is the aspect of mind that is the ego sense, which does not stop or settle down.* It won't do that! It is the aspect of mind that is known in India as the 'monkey mind' and is by its nature very active. In fact, we need it to be very active. Yet we can be aware of its activity yet still in touch with the natural mind (*citta* in both Sanskrit and Pali) – the one that can settle.

I know there are many traditions that encourage long

*The Wikipedia article online about ahamkara *is particularly interesting. See https://en.wikipedia.org/wiki/Ahamkara. For more about* citta, *see the note on p. 108.*

hours of sitting, which is admirable, but if the spine slumps and the head drops forward, then doesn't the mind become very active? Then we have to force it back to the breath or look at where it goes, which we can also do throughout our daily life if we take a little time to contemplate.

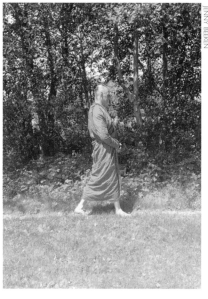

I have just spent almost a year living at Cittaviveka – Chithurst Buddhist Monastery in Sussex, England. The practice there on retreats and on full and half moon days was to sit for forty-five minutes, then practice walking meditation for forty-five minutes (see below), and then sit again for forty-five minutes. You were invited to do this from 7.30 pm to 3.30 am and beyond on Moon nights.

I only managed to stay awake until 10.30 pm, except on New Year's Eve, when there was the incentive of hot chocolate, dark chocolate and crystallized ginger! These treats came after chanting around the stupa at midnight having placed paper, written with all you wanted to let go of from the old year on the fire burning there, keeping what you would like to bring into the new year. It was a most appropriate and splendid way to spend New Year's Eve – with the sound of distant fireworks to complete the picture!

Walking Meditation

Going for a walk can be a wonderful practice in mindfulness if you are first aware of your body: aware of how your feet engage

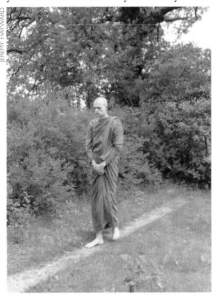

with the ground underneath you, then how that lengthens your legs up through your hips to your spine and so gives a rhythm to your breath coming in and going out. Yet walking meditation as the Buddha taught it is very different from going for a walk. It is more settling on the mind, to encourage sitting afterwards.

Find a reasonably flat straight path of maybe twenty or thirty steps and stand in *tadasana*, mountain posture (see p. 58) at one end of the path. Bring your awareness to your breathing and slowly, gently walk the paces to the end. Pause, turn and walk back, keeping your gaze down and ahead of you, aware of the Earth underneath you, the contact of your feet with the earth and the length up through your legs to your spine. When you pause, feel the feet firm on the ground, the legs connecting through the hips to the spine, the shoulders winging out to the sides and the neck lengthening, so that your head sits up and back on the atlas/axis vertebrae (as described in chapter 2, p. 34)

Continue for at least ten minutes, extending the time with

practice. It is especially helpful when the mind feels too busy to sit. There are a few monks and practitioners at Chithurst who do walking meditation much of the time rather than sitting.

The Buddha taught that we be constantly aware of the breathing coming in and going out without altering it in any way. There is a lot to be said for not trying to change how you breathe, because bringing your full attention to the movement of the breath through the body does change it naturally and gently over time and with regular practice. The inhalation and exhalation will find their normal rhythm with a natural pause at the end of the exhalation. In my understanding the Buddha taught mindfulness of breathing in order to deal with the mind and become aware of the different aspects of the mind.

Nirvana

Alistair Shearer, in his examination of the meaning of *pranayama*, quoted on p. 81, says that one translation of *nirvana* is 'no breath'. When the mind and body relax in the mindfulness of breathing practice or after specific *pranayama* practice you can sometimes find as you go on sitting with the effects of all these practices, that the inhalation and exhalation settle down almost as if they are not there. You cannot make this happen by effort of will – it's a quietening of whole self. Rather, it can arise when you let it be. It is a natural outcome of all these practices, a stillness that can be enjoyed and appreciated but not held onto – yet remembered in our everyday life and in day-to-day breathing.

Before or after the exercise that follows, it can be very helpful to chant or say a prayer in invocation. See the Divine Abidings chant at the end of the book for an example.

The Buddha's Mindfulness of Breathing

The following is an adaptation of the Buddha's Mindfulness of Breathing Sutta (given about 2,500 years ago to his monastic community) for twenty-first century civilization.

Sitting with the spine upright on a chair or on the ground, as described in the posture chapter, become aware of breathing in.

Become aware of breathing out as you lengthen down through the tailbone. Breathing in, breathing out, feel the spine lengthen up to the crown. Be aware that your breathing deepens as you do this, without you making it do so.

Feel as the spine comes up through the shoulders that the shoulders open out, the heart lifts and the collarbones wing out.

Breathing in, breathing out, become aware of bodily formations (see pp 107-8) where the body tightens around the head, the jaw, the tongue, the neck and shoulders.

As you breathe out, gradually relax all those tight areas. This may take several breaths.

Keep the lengthening forward and up of the spine.

Feel how the breath settles into a rhythm, tending to lengthen without you making it do so, for several breaths. The Buddha termed this 'long inhalation, long exhalation'.

Then your breath will naturally shorten to a rhythm that would then be your normal rate of breathing. The Buddha termed this 'short inhalation, short exhalation'.

Now be aware of the mental formations, also termed mental objects or mental transitions. These are the topics that the day-to-day mind gets preoccupied with but can constantly be changing.

Breathing in, breathing out, let go of those mental formations. You can then be aware of the natural mind, the heart-mind,* and aware of breathing in, breathing out. This is the part of the mind and heart that can settle.

Continuing breathing in and breathing out. Gladden the heart, the mind.

Breathing in, breathing out, focus the heart, the mind.

Breathing in, breathing out, settle the heart, the mind (*samadhi*).

Breathing in, breathing out, liberate the heart, the mind (*nirvana*).

Breathing in, breathing out, contemplate impermanence and uncertainty.

Breathing in, breathing out, contemplate relinquishment.

Breathing in, breathing out, let go, let go, let go.

Breathing in, breathing out, gradually come out of your meditation.

The Buddha gave the Sanskrit and Pali word 'citta' here, which Luang Por Sucitto of Cittaviveka Monastery translates as heart, mind, awareness. The ancient texts do not differentiate so much between heart and mind: they are generally interchangeable in the Buddha's teaching!

Recent research shows many more neural pathways from the heart to the mind than from the mind to the heart, perhaps confirming that connection for the scientifically minded? It can be very helpful in meditation to bring your whole awareness to the heart area as you breathe in and breathe out.

Chapter 8 : Healing through Breathing

'The practice of yoga is the commitment to become established in the state of freedom.
'The practice of yoga will be firmly rooted when it is maintained consistently and with dedication over a long period.'
Patanjali's Sutras 1.13 and 1.14,
in Alistair Shearer's translation.

'Healing is different from curing or fixing.'
Leslie Kaminoff

Breathing that Relieves Dis-ease

HEALING IS a release of old holding patterns – *samskaras* in Sanskrit or *sankara* in Pali – and needs to come from within the individual person at the level of the natural self, mind, heart – the *citta*. *Citta* is also called consciousness by Sri B. K. S. Iyengar. Disease is best seen as lack of ease, dis-ease.

Yoga practice at all levels has a profound effect on the whole body, mind, breath, heart and soul. However, it needs to be practised regularly in a relaxed but very precise, firm way to relieve any dis-ease at any level in the system. This needs a lot of insight and dedication in the yoga teacher and practitioner, and is very individual to the person as well as to the nature of the disease – and of course to the expertise and awareness of the teacher. It usually needs one-to-one attention, and therefore no claims can be made as to the effects of the practice: only time and perseverance will bring about sure, long lasting results.

Since I began this book I have continued to study Iain McGilchrist's massive work on the two sides of the brain mentioned on p. 89, as it is so relevant to the breath. I have felt, lying down in *savasana*, that when the breath can come in through the left nostril, I feel the right side of the brain relax as though the breath could spread out more into the right side of the skull. This feels as though it frees up the aspect of the mind that can encompass the world around – just as the bird (remembering the predator and prey viewpoints pn pp 64-7) is aware of what is going on around him or her. The whole left side of the body then felt it could relax more, especially down through the sacrum.

Repeating this through the right nostril I could then connect over to the left side of the brain. I felt I could feel the more focused awareness of that side and realized the truth of Albert Einstein's statement on p. 90 that we have given more prominence to that focus.

Doing this enabled me to find more balance in the two very different hemispheres of the brain and life. If we could keep this awareness we could see how these two aspects of mind come into conflict within ourselves and that would free us to be aware of where our priorities lie and so trust our more intuitive nature.

This awareness of the breath moving through the nostrils and connecting to the hemispheres of the brain is at the level of the more subtle breath body, called in Sanskrit the *prana-maya-kosa*. Here, *prana* is life force, *maya* is illusion (in yoga and in the Buddha's teaching, anything that is subject to change is illusion) and *kosa* is a layering. Usually in our current stage of civilization we have only awareness of the denser *ana-maya-kosa* – where ana means of food. In short, we have built a dense physical body from the food we eat.

As we refine our breathing we become aware of this more subtle body which moves through the physical and is more to do with our energy. As we become more aware of our breathing and thus to a more subtle awareness of our body, it will connect us to the planet Earth and what is happening to it.

The movement of the Ida and Pingala through the body as the breath comes through the left nostril then spirals across into the right hemisphere of the brain, travels across to left and spirals out through the right nostril reminds me of the spiralling drawings on the very ancient prehistoric stones at the Newgrange in Ireland (as in the picture below). Is it possible that the ancient civilization that built these amazing,enduring monuments could have more awareness than we do now of the earth's energy?

Can we regain that awareness by becoming aware of how our breath moves through our body – and will that put us more in touch with the earth's energy to give us more care and realization of the effects we are having on the natural world? All the challenges that I mentioned in the Introduction to this book may have some roots in the simple process of how we breathe and the awareness that goes with it.

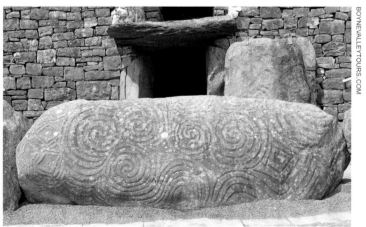

Engraved spirals on the ancient stones at Newgrange, in Ireland

Personal Experience

I feel my own awareness has been increased by reducing how much I breathe through my mouth. It has increased the sensitivity of the wider open nostril to the opposite sphere of the brain. This unexpected experience has led me to understand how the breath moves with the energy channels in the body at a subtle level. It was stated above that in yoga there are said to be 72,000 energy channels in the body. However, there are three main ones: the *ida* feminine energy-channel moves from the left side of the base of the spine and spirals up around the spine, going through the left nostril, crossing over at the bridge of the nose to the right hemisphere of the brain. The *pingala* masculine energy channel moves from the right side of the base of the spine and spirals up around the spine going through the right nostril, crossing over at the bridge of the nose to the left hemisphere of the brain. This spiral of the *ida* and *pingala* around the spine stimulates the *sushumna nadi* to move straight up through the centre of the spine, clearing and cleansing as it goes.

I think from this it is clear that to force the process by blocking one nostril to breathe through the other is not going with that spiral of the *ida* energy from the left to the right and the *pingala* energy from the right to the left. I have felt this but never really experienced it in this way until recently. The revelation shows the need we really to be in touch with our own bodies and our breath and to trust what the body needs to do. It also makes me realize the depth and subtlety of the very ancient practice of yoga.

If we can find more of a balance between the hemispheres of the brain and their connection to our bodies, I believe this might enable us to recreate that balance in nature. Then we would then really address climate change and the threatened extinction of species, including ourselves.

I have experienced tremendous results in myself and seen them in others who have a dedicated and consistent practice – conditions such as deterioration in the spine and neck being relieved, mental states of anxiety and depression being managed. There is much research going on about the benefits of both yoga and good breathing, but the research is often ignored by the orthodox medical profession as it is very difficult to have a 'control group' and there aren't a lot of commercial incentives attached to it. So I am here going to give examples of people I know in person, and people's own testimonials – all who have benefited from particular changes in their breathing habits or have adopted a new way of breathing for them.

In my own case, breathing practice lifts me out of depression and anxiety, helps me sleep, and stimulates my mind into writing books. Once – indeed five times over! – I ran courses for management teams at IBM. Several participants said it was the toughest management course they had been on. Afterwards a group continued in a weekly class. It was very brave of them. They were almost all men, all with hypertension – that is, high blood pressure and other connected dis-ease. All fifteen of them habitually held their breath. To help heal this I

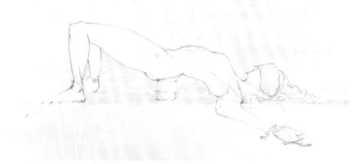

Bridge pose, with support under the sacrum and and an eye-pad or scarf across the eyes and forehead

asked them to start the class in a ten-minute supported Bridge pose – *setu-bandha savangasana*.

They then went through a series of basic standing, sitting and lying postures for an hour with me, with awareness of breathing, including awareness of their tendency to hold the breath in, followed by twenty minutes of relaxation and awareness of breathing and how it lengthens and deepens when you give it full attention.

Many of those who then engaged in a regular practice of yoga and awareness of breathing (when they gave a thought to it in their busy day), found that their blood pressure went down over time to a more normal level. If they were able to continue this practice over time, there would be a healing of the underlying causes of hypertension and a shift in their lives and themselves.

My sister, who has been asthmatic for many years, using inhalers daily, consciously adopted the '5.5' resonant breathing and this has reduced the use of her inhaler considerably .

What follow are the personal stories of some I know to have benefitted from breathing practice. First, my publisher, Colum Hayward, writes:

'This book had a strange birthing moment when I was sitting outside a café in Barnes, south-west London, with Jenny. I'd described some chronic conditions that were troubling my health, and she surprised me by insisting that I lean forward, as if onto the table, right there in the street as people walked past. Then she led me in a practice, unforgettably telling me, as the incoming air filled the back of my lungs, to remember that through the breath I was connected to everything else in the Universe.

'Sometimes instructions that you have heard before, in one extraordinary moment take on particular significance. In that moment I really was one – absolutely one – with all life. The feeling is beyond describing as that kind of connection does not come from the part of us that knows words. That was the power of it:

a knowledge that absolutely nothing but illusion keeps us apart from one another – and apart from rocks, and stones, and trees.'

Next are stories of students of mine.

'A year ago I attended a course in *pranayama*. I thought it would be a good way to get back to yoga practice after a break of a few years. It was a short course – four classes, each of one and a half hours – where we learned some basic breathing techniques based on *ujjayi* breathing. Already at the first occasion I noticed that the headache I had when we started was gone when the class was over. I was a bit familiar to *Ujjayi* breathing since I learned it when I was practising ashtanga yoga earlier in life, but I had never really before given myself the opportunity to put my full attention on just the breathing part. Now I had to do that and I was amazed by how it affected my body and my mind. I felt like I gained access to my own strength and became centered in myself. It actually brought me more self confidence.

'I also realized that a feeling of tiredness can be relieved by sitting and actively breathing for a while. And it gave me better sleep. I remember asking the teacher for the course why there tends to be so much focus on the asanas in yoga practice when this must be the thing! Today I do *pranayama* regularly – sometimes together with asanas, sometimes as a separate practice, and I am still surpriced and most of all very grateful for the positive effects it brings. When I get headaches today I sit down and do breathing exercises for ten to fifteen minutes and almost every time the pain leaves.'   *Johanna Bergsten*

'Breath practice helps me identify areas of tension in both body and mind. If I can focus on these points, give them the individual love they deserve, I am often rewarded with a revelation, life learning point or a release of emotion. Emotional release is usually associated with the past and allows me to incrementally make peace with some difficult experiences. I use breath practice to help with sleeplessness – and bizarrely, at the other end of the spectrum, sitting in lay-bys trying to wake up and stay awake at the wheel. Sometimes I practice with my son. It seems to help teenage life!'   *Helen Thomas*

'Simply having an invitation to notice the breath, to notice the body, is powerful for me, bringing a sense of grounding and reconnection with myself which may have become over-looked – a more holistic mindfulness – embracing all aspects of the self.'   *Liz Mitchell*

'Breathing is not a practice that I gave great importance to but I am becoming more and more aware of its importance. It is something I took for granted because it is automatic, but by becoming aware of it everything suddenly changes. The focus on the breath lightens my body and my mind and allows me to perceive what is real and not what the narrative or conver-sation in my head tells me. So breathing takes me to the truth, to an uncluttered perception of what is. At the end of the breath, when there is a still point or pause and when the whole body settles, there is an expanse which allows everything to empty and it feels safe. Perhaps it's a point of surrender which is actually reassuring rather than terrifying.' *Catharine Ireland*

'My experience of the breath is of its amazing powers to re-lease tension and focus the mind. As a child and young adult, I was familiar with the expression, "take a deep breath", when things were challenging. However, I never really noticed what that breath was actually doing to my body. It was only through my practice of yoga that I was able to use the breath to release tension in my body. I also find that it can help me go deeper into a pose without force, just a release of tension that may be getting in the way. In meditation, I use the breath to focus my mind. Usually by focusing on the movement of the ribs and the diaphragm. My acknowledgment of the breath came a lot later than it should have done but is now completely intertwined with my yoga practice and my daily life.' *Sonja Balmer*

'During the Covid pandemic, both I and my husband Jon, who is also a yoga teacher, were diagnosed with cancer on the very same day. As we'd been feeling fit and well, this came as a tremendous shock. Our practice of meditation and mindful breathing helped us through a difficult journey. During a long wait for diagnostic procedures, mindful breathing became an anchor steadying my mind, my overactive thoughts. Acknowledging and naming the emotions as they surfaced became most helpful and settling, along with simply watching and witnessing the breath.

'Jon and I both had surgery during late summer and without a doubt our practice helped with the healing process. It also helped me to cope with the sessions of radiotherapy which were to follow during lockdown. On returning to teaching, it was heartwarming to hear that two of my students had also found enormous benefit from mindful breathing whilst experiencing high levels of anxiety due to hospital procedures.

'Mindful breathing and meditation will continue to be a large part of my practice, my teaching and my life.' *Mari Dixon*

Chanting and Mindfulness

My students also contributed thoughts about how they had been helped forward by chanting, and by mindfulness practice.

'I was a reluctant "chanter" when I was first introduced to it. Embarrassment and fear of "not knowing the words" kept me silent. However, once I grew in confidence, I really enjoyed it. Chanting always feels joyful and lifts my mood. I love noticing the vibrations of sound through the body and how this can not only settle the mind but also create a feeling of being connected.'

Sonja Balmer

'Chanting has become part of my daily practice and life. Each morning I chant various chants. This focuses me and connects me inwardly and leads me into my asana practice.

'During the day while walking and if my mind is preoccupied with thoughts chanting brings me to the present, aware of my breathing, aware of my surroundings.

'I discovered recently how chanting can help me fall asleep, especially when I have not had sufficient unwinding time before going to bed. Chanting Patanjali's opening lines of the Yoga Sutras (1 : 2-4), in Sanskrit, a few times, very quickly lulls me to sleep. The words are so appropriate and speak to the busy mind. I am also reminded of the Buddhist tradition of taking care what you think about when going to sleep as it may be your final sleep :

Yogah cittavrtti nirodhah
tada drastuh svarupe avasthanam
vritti sarupyam itaratra

'In Alastair Shearer's translation:
Yoga is the settling of the mind into silence.
When the mind is settled we are established
in our essential nature which is unbounded consciousness.
Our essential nature is usually overshadowed by the activities of the mind.'   *Chris Wyeth*

'I was "practising" mindfulness, before I knew it had a name or was a thing. One of my favourite ways to unwind is to go walking in the beautiful countryside that I am lucky enough to live in. I spend these walks 'noticing'. Birdsong, flowers, trees, the changing of the seasons. Quite often, not a single other thought will enter my mind. Just the here and now and an appreciation of nature's beauty.'   *Sonja Balmer*

'Sitting outside on the grass or it could be a wall, a rock, on a beach, wherever.

'Perhaps I might be standing, barefoot, feet in touch with the ground, the Earth.

'And breathe.

'My outer sight is stalled by eyelids closed, breath goes a little "do-lally" with the slightest attention, but then it finds a gentle deeper rhythm, and in turn my mind begins to let go and release its tightness.

'Hearing is on "peripheral" and in breathing I feel totally at one and thankful to the flora around me, for as I inhale I am taking in the given gift of oxygen from the greenery around me, and in return on my exhalation of carbon dioxide I can know for sure it will be glady absorbed by the trees and plants in return.

'So I have a connection to flora above ground through my breath, but there's another connection ... roots, as sitting or standing upon the Earth, I am sending my 'roots' deep down, through any parts of myself in contact with the ground.

'As my "roots" descend they connect to the roots of all the flora roots around me, in the cool, dark earth, I'm grounded and connected, and it is that that brings a steadying and a settling of my anxious mind and my breath can find a peaceful rhythm connected to Nature.'

Murray Nettle

All these ideas, instructions and practices are of course not just for ourselves but for passing on in teaching formally or informally, but they also help us to be a facilitator for healing others in some way or another way: maybe by sending thoughts, best wishes, condolences, light, love, starlight or one of the Buddha's invocations, such as the chant on the next pages.

The Divine Abidings Chant

I will abide, pervading one quarter of the world with a heart imbued with loving kindness,

Likewise the second, likewise the third, likewise the fourth,

So above and below, around and everywhere. And to all as to myself.

I will abide pervading an all-encompassing world with a heart imbued with loving kindness,

Abundant, Immeasurable, exalted, without hostility and without ill will.

I will abide pervading one quarter of the world with a heart imbued with compassion,

Likewise the second, likewise the third, likewise the fourth,

So above and below, around and everywhere and to all as to myself.

I will abide pervading an all-encompassing world with a heart imbued with compassion

Abundant, Immeasurable, exalted, without hostility and without ill will.

I will abide pervading one quarter of the world with a heart imbued with gladness,

Likewise the second, likewise the third, likewise the fourth,

So above and below around and everywhere and to all as to myself.

[continues]

> I will abide pervading an all-encompassing world with a heart imbued with gladness,
> Abundant, immeasurable, exalted, without hostility and without ill will..
>
> I will abide pervading one quarter of the world with a heart imbued with equanimity,
> Likewise the second, likewise the third, likewise the fourth.
>
> So above and below and around and everywhere and to all as to myself.
> I will abide pervading an all-encompassing world with a heart imbued with equanimity,
>
> Abundant, immeasurable, exalted without hostility and without ill will.

Buddha's words are a profound accompaniment to awareness of breathing.

The Lord Jesus Christ, the Great Healer, said:

'Love another, as I have loved you'

Maybe that is the ultimate healing? 'Respiration' when split into its components is 're-inspire-ation'. 'Inspire' means 'in-spirit'. The English word 'spirit' comes from the Latin 'spiritus' meaning 'breath' so we come round in a circle here. 'Re' implies we return to it, revisit. So respiration is 'return to the spirit' or connect to the spirit or your source in whatever way is real for you. Each time we breathe – inspiration and expiration – we re-inspire ourselves.

FURTHER STUDY

Ancient texts

THE YOGA SUTRAS OF PATANJALI, translated by Alistair Shearer (Rider, 2002)

THE TEN PRINICPAL UPANISHADS, translated by Shree Purohit Swami and W. B. Yeats (Faber and Faber, 1970)

THE HATHA YOGA PRADIPIKA with commentary by Swami Saraswati (Yoga Publications Trust)

THE MINDFULNESS OF BREATHING SUTTA – available from Amaravati. org/teachings/chanting

Yoga books cited or recommended

LIGHT ON PRANAYAMA, by B.K.S Iyengar (Thoresens, 1981)

AWAKENING THE SPINE, by Vanda Scaravelli. (Aquarian Press, 1995)

NOTES ON YOGA: THE LEGACY OF VANDA SCARAVELLI, by Diane Long and Sophy Hoare (YogaWords, 2016)

STANDING, SITTING, WALKING, RUNNING, by Jenny Beeken (Polair Publishing, 2016)

THE YOGA OF EATING, by Charles Eisenstein (New Trends, 2003)

DANCING THE FLAME OF LIFE, by Dona Holleman (YogaWords, 2015)

Books on breathing

BREATH, by James Nestor (Penguin, 2020)

THE BREATHING CURE, by Patrick McKeown (OxyAt Books, 2021)

THE TAO OF NATURAL BREATHING, by Dennis Lewis (Shambala, 1996)

On Mind and Brain

THE MASTER AND HIS EMISSARY, by Iain McGilchrist. New expanded edition (Yale, 2019); also, his TED talk, 'The Divided Brain and theSearch for Meaning', at https://www.youtube.com/watch?v=vk-mYzbwrufg

Where to find a yoga teacher

WWW.INNERYOGA.ORG.UK has a list of trained teachers and teacher training courses. Write to Danielle@inneryoga.org.uk for further information.

WWW.INNERYOGALONDON.CO.UK runs classes, workshops and a teacher training course

WWW.DIANELONGYOGA.COM gives Diane Long's schedule for teaching and recommendations of teachers

Victor van Kooten and Angela Farmer, www.victor-angela.com, run courses in Greece.

On Facebook: Scaravelli Inspired Yoga gives contacts of yoga teachers

Where to find the Buddha's Theravada Monasteries

The monastery at which I lived on retreat was Chithurst Buddhist Monastery in Sussex, England, www.cittaviveka.org

Jenny Beeken

Jenny (jennybeeken48@gmail.com) runs posture, breathing, mindfulness and meditation classes, courses, retreat days and residential holidays/retreats and Zoom classes, as well as meditation and days relating to the Celtic calendar.

INDEX